CONTENTS

4

CANDY BAR FUSION ICE CREAM

Heath Bar Soft Serve Ice Cream

Servings: 6
Cooking Time: 35 Minutes
Ingredients:
- 2 cups heavy cream
- 1 cup milk
- 3/4 cup sugar
- 1 Tbs. vanilla extract
- 1 cup sliced Bananas
- 2 Heath Bar Candy Bars.

Directions:
1. Refer to note at the beginning of the chapter about freezing bowl.
2. Place the milk & cream in a bowl. Mix together until well combined. Use a whisk to mix in the sugar. Continue to whisking 4 minutes until sugar dissolves. Then mix in the vanilla extract.
3. Place all the ingredients in a food processor or blender, and puree.
4. Pour ingredients into ice cream maker. Let it churn for 25 minutes.
5. Serve immediately.

Charleston Chew Soft Serve Ice Cream

Servings: 6
Cooking Time: 35 Minutes
Ingredients:
- 2 cups heavy cream
- 1 cup milk
- 3/4 cup sugar
- 1 Tbs. vanilla extract
- 1 cup sliced Bananas
- 2 Charleston Chew Candy Bars.

Directions:
1. Refer to note at the beginning of the chapter about freezing bowl.
2. Place the milk & cream in a bowl. Mix together until well combined. Use a whisk to mix in the sugar. Continue to whisking 4 minutes until sugar dissolves. Then mix in the vanilla extract.
3. Place all the ingredients in a food processor or blender, and puree.

4. Pour ingredients into ice cream maker. Let it churn for 25 minutes.

Zero Soft Serve Ice Cream

Servings: 6
Cooking Time: 35 Minutes
Ingredients:
- 2 cups heavy cream
- 1 cup milk
- 3/4 cup sugar
- 1 Tbs. vanilla extract
- 1 cup sliced Bananas
- 2 Zero Candy Bars.

Directions:
1. Refer to note at the beginning of the chapter about freezing bowl.
2. Place the milk & cream in a bowl. Mix together until well combined. Use a whisk to mix in the sugar. Continue to whisking 4 minutes until sugar dissolves. Then mix in the vanilla extract.
3. Place all the ingredients in a food processor or blender, and puree.
4. Pour ingredients into ice cream maker. Let it churn for 25 minutes.

Sky Bar Soft Serve Ice Cream

Servings: 6
Cooking Time: 35 Minutes
Ingredients:
- 2 cups heavy cream
- 1 cup milk
- 3/4 cup sugar
- 1 Tbs. vanilla extract
- 1 cup sliced Bananas
- 2 Sky Bar Candy Bars.

Directions:
1. Refer to note at the beginning of the chapter about freezing bowl.
2. Place the milk & cream in a bowl. Mix together until well combined. Use a whisk to mix in the sugar. Continue to whisking 4 minutes until sugar dissolves. Then mix in the vanilla extract.

3. Place all the ingredients in a food processor or blender, and puree.
4. Pour ingredients into ice cream maker. Let it churn for 25 minutes.
5. Serve immediately.

Twix Soft Serve Ice Cream

Servings: 6
Cooking Time: 35 Minutes
Ingredients:
- 2 cups heavy cream
- 1 cup milk
- 3/4 cup sugar
- 1 Tbs. vanilla extract
- 1 cup sliced Bananas
- 4 Twix Candy Bars.

Directions:
1. Refer to note at the beginning of the chapter about freezing bowl.
2. Place the milk & cream in a bowl. Mix together until well combined. Use a whisk to mix in the sugar. Continue to whisking 4 minutes until sugar dissolves. Then mix in the vanilla extract.
3. Place all the ingredients in a food processor or blender, and puree.
4. Pour ingredients into ice cream maker. Let it churn for 25 minutes.

Hershey Bar Soft Serve Ice Cream

Servings: 6
Cooking Time: 35 Minutes
Ingredients:
- 2 cups heavy cream
- 1 cup milk
- 3/4 cup sugar
- 1 Tbs. vanilla extract
- 1 cup sliced Bananas
- 2 Hershey Bar Candy Bars.

Directions:
1. Refer to note at the beginning of the chapter about freezing bowl.
2. Place the milk & cream in a bowl. Mix together until well combined. Use a whisk to mix in the sugar.

Continue to whisking 4 minutes until sugar dissolves. Then mix in the vanilla extract.
3. Place all the ingredients in a food processor or blender, and puree.
4. Pour ingredients into ice cream maker. Let it churn for 25 minutes.
5. Serve immediately.

Take 5 Soft Serve Ice Cream

Servings: 6
Cooking Time: 35 Minutes
Ingredients:
- 2 cups heavy cream
- 1 cup milk
- 3/4 cup sugar
- 1 Tbs. vanilla extract
- 1 cup sliced Bananas
- 2 Take 5 Candy Bars.

Directions:
1. Refer to note at the beginning of the chapter about freezing bowl.
2. Place the milk & cream in a bowl. Mix together until well combined. Use a whisk to mix in the sugar. Continue to whisking 4 minutes until sugar dissolves. Then mix in the vanilla extract.
3. Place all the ingredients in a food processor or blender, and puree.
4. Pour ingredients into ice cream maker. Let it churn for 25 minutes.
5. Serve immediately.

Snickers Soft Serve Ice Cream

Servings: 6
Cooking Time: 35 Minutes
Ingredients:
- 2 cups heavy cream
- 1 cup milk
- 3/4 cup sugar
- 1 Tbs. vanilla extract
- 1 cup sliced Bananas
- 2 Snickers Candy Bars.

Directions:
1. Refer to note at the beginning of the chapter about freezing bowl.

2. Place the milk & cream in a bowl. Mix together until well combined. Use a whisk to mix in the sugar. Continue to whisking 4 minutes until sugar dissolves. Then mix in the vanilla extract.
3. Place all the ingredients in a food processor or blender, and puree.
4. Pour ingredients into ice cream maker. Let it churn for 25 minutes.

Butterfinger Soft Serve Ice Cream

Servings: 6
Cooking Time: 35 Minutes
Ingredients:
- 2 cups heavy cream
- 1 cup milk
- 3/4 cup sugar
- 1 Tbs. vanilla extract
- 1 cup sliced Bananas
- 2 Butterfinger Candy Bars.

Directions:
1. Refer to note at the beginning of the chapter about freezing bowl.
2. Place the milk & cream in a bowl. Mix together until well combined. Use a whisk to mix in the sugar. Continue to whisking 4 minutes until sugar dissolves. Then mix in the vanilla extract.
3. Place all the ingredients in a food processor or blender, and puree.
4. Pour ingredients into ice cream maker. Let it churn for 25 minutes.
5. Serve immediately.

Mr. Goodbar Soft Serve Ice Cream

Servings: 6
Cooking Time: 35 Minutes
Ingredients:
- 2 cups heavy cream
- 1 cup milk
- 3/4 cup sugar
- 1 Tbs. vanilla extract
- 1 cup sliced Bananas
- 2 Mr. Goodbar Candy Bars.

Directions:

1. Refer to note at the beginning of the chapter about freezing bowl.
2. Place the milk & cream in a bowl. Mix together until well combined. Use a whisk to mix in the sugar. Continue to whisking 4 minutes until sugar dissolves. Then mix in the vanilla extract.
3. Place all the ingredients in a food processor or blender, and puree.
4. Pour ingredients into ice cream maker. Let it churn for 25 minutes.
5. Serve immediately.

Pay Day Soft Serve Ice Cream

Servings: 6
Cooking Time: 35 Minutes
Ingredients:
- 2 cups heavy cream
- 1 cup milk
- 3/4 cup sugar
- 1 Tbs. vanilla extract
- 1 cup sliced Bananas
- 2 Pay Day Candy Bars.

Directions:
1. Refer to note at the beginning of the chapter about freezing bowl.
2. Place the milk & cream in a bowl. Mix together until well combined. Use a whisk to mix in the sugar. Continue to whisking 4 minutes until sugar dissolves. Then mix in the vanilla extract.
3. Place all the ingredients in a food processor or blender, and puree.
4. Pour ingredients into ice cream maker. Let it churn for 25 minutes.

3 Musketeers Soft Serve Ice Cream

Servings: 6
Cooking Time: 35 Minutes
Ingredients:
- 2 cups heavy cream
- 1 cup milk
- 3/4 cup sugar
- 1 Tbs. vanilla extract
- 1 cup sliced Bananas
- 2 3 Musketeers Candy Bars.

Directions:

1. Refer to note at the beginning of the chapter about freezing bowl.
2. Place the milk & cream in a bowl. Mix together until well combined. Use a whisk to mix in the sugar. Continue to whisking 4 minutes until sugar dissolves. Then mix in the vanilla extract.
3. Place all the ingredients in a food processor or blender, and puree.
4. Pour ingredients into ice cream maker. Let it churn for 25 minutes.

Directions:

1. Refer to note at the beginning of the chapter about freezing bowl.
2. Place the milk & cream in a bowl. Mix together until well combined. Use a whisk to mix in the sugar. Continue to whisking 4 minutes until sugar dissolves. Then mix in the vanilla extract.
3. Place all the ingredients in a food processor or blender, and puree.
4. Pour ingredients into ice cream maker. Let it churn for 25 minutes.

Mounds Soft Serve Ice Cream

Servings: 6
Cooking Time: 35 Minutes
Ingredients:

- 2 cups heavy cream
- 1 cup milk
- 3/4 cup sugar
- 1 Tbs. vanilla extract
- 1 cup sliced Bananas
- 2 Mounds Candy Bars.

Directions:

1. Refer to note at the beginning of the chapter about freezing bowl.
2. Place the milk & cream in a bowl. Mix together until well combined. Use a whisk to mix in the sugar. Continue to whisking 4 minutes until sugar dissolves. Then mix in the vanilla extract.
3. Place all the ingredients in a food processor or blender, and puree.
4. Pour ingredients into ice cream maker. Let it churn for 25 minutes.

Mars Bar Soft Serve Ice Cream

Servings: 6
Cooking Time: 35 Minutes
Ingredients:

- 2 cups heavy cream
- 1 cup milk
- 3/4 cup sugar
- 1 Tbs. vanilla extract
- 1 cup sliced Bananas
- 2 Mars Bar Candy Bars.

Directions:

1. Refer to note at the beginning of the chapter about freezing bowl.
2. Place the milk & cream in a bowl. Mix together until well combined. Use a whisk to mix in the sugar. Continue to whisking 4 minutes until sugar dissolves. Then mix in the vanilla extract.
3. Place all the ingredients in a food processor or blender, and puree.
4. Pour ingredients into ice cream maker. Let it churn for 25 minutes.

Krackel Soft Serve Ice Cream

Servings: 6
Cooking Time: 35 Minutes
Ingredients:

- 2 cups heavy cream
- 1 cup milk
- 3/4 cup sugar
- 1 Tbs. vanilla extract
- 1 cup sliced Bananas
- 2 Krackel Candy Bars.

Skor Bar Soft Serve Ice Cream

Servings: 6
Cooking Time: 35 Minutes
Ingredients:

- 2 cups heavy cream
- 1 cup milk
- 3/4 cup sugar
- 1 Tbs. vanilla extract
- 1 cup sliced Bananas
- 2 Skor Bar Candy Bars.

Directions:

1. Refer to note at the beginning of the chapter about freezing bowl.
2. Place the milk & cream in a bowl. Mix together until well combined. Use a whisk to mix in the sugar. Continue to whisking 4 minutes until sugar dissolves. Then mix in the vanilla extract.
3. Place all the ingredients in a food processor or blender, and puree.
4. Pour ingredients into ice cream maker. Let it churn for 25 minutes.
5. Serve immediately.

Milky Way Soft Serve Ice Cream

Servings: 6
Cooking Time: 35 Minutes
Ingredients:

- 2 cups heavy cream
- 1 cup milk
- 3/4 cup sugar
- 1 Tbs. vanilla extract
- 1 cup sliced Bananas
- 2 Milky Way Candy Bars.

Directions:

1. Refer to note at the beginning of the chapter about freezing bowl.
2. Place the milk & cream in a bowl. Mix together until well combined. Use a whisk to mix in the sugar. Continue to whisking 4 minutes until sugar dissolves. Then mix in the vanilla extract.
3. Place all the ingredients in a food processor or blender, and puree.
4. Pour ingredients into ice cream maker. Let it churn for 25 minutes.

Almond Joy Soft Serve Ice Cream

Servings: 6
Cooking Time: 35 Minutes
Ingredients:

- 2 cups heavy cream
- 1 cup milk
- 3/4 cup sugar
- 1 Tbs. vanilla extract
- 1 cup sliced Bananas

- 2 Almond Joy Candy Bars.

Directions:

1. Refer to note at the beginning of the chapter about freezing bowl.
2. Place the milk & cream in a bowl. Mix together until well combined. Use a whisk to mix in the sugar. Continue to whisking 4 minutes until sugar dissolves. Then mix in the vanilla extract.
3. Place all the ingredients in a food processor or blender, and puree.
4. Pour ingredients into ice cream maker. Let it churn for 25 minutes.
5. Serve immediately.

Kit Kat Soft Serve Ice Cream

Servings: 6
Cooking Time: 35 Minutes
Ingredients:

- 2 cups heavy cream
- 1 cup milk
- 3/4 cup sugar
- 1 Tbs. vanilla extract
- 1 cup sliced Bananas
- 2 Kit Kat Candy Bars.

Directions:

1. Refer to note at the beginning of the chapter about freezing bowl.
2. Place the milk & cream in a bowl. Mix together until well combined. Use a whisk to mix in the sugar. Continue to whisking 4 minutes until sugar dissolves. Then mix in the vanilla extract.
3. Place all the ingredients in a food processor or blender, and puree.
4. Pour ingredients into ice cream maker. Let it churn for 25 minutes.

Caramello Dreamin Soft Serve Ice Cream

Servings: 6
Cooking Time: 35 Minutes
Ingredients:

- 2 cups heavy cream
- 1 cup milk
- 3/4 cup sugar
- 1 Tbs. vanilla extract

- 1 cup sliced Bananas
- 2 Caramello Candy Bars.

Directions:

1. Refer to note at the beginning of the chapter about freezing bowl.
2. Place the milk & cream in a bowl. Mix together until well combined. Use a whisk to mix in the sugar. Continue to whisking 4 minutes until sugar dissolves. Then mix in the vanilla extract.
3. Place all the ingredients in a food processor or blender, and puree.
4. Pour ingredients into ice cream maker. Let it churn for 25 minutes.
5. Serve immediately.

Baby Ruth Soft Serve Ice Cream

Servings: 6
Cooking Time: 35 Minutes
Ingredients:

- 2 cups heavy cream
- 1 cup milk
- 3/4 cup sugar
- 1 Tbs. vanilla extract
- 1 cup sliced Bananas
- 2 Baby Ruth Candy Bars.

Directions:

1. Refer to note at the beginning of the chapter about freezing bowl.
2. Place the milk & cream in a bowl. Mix together until well combined. Use a whisk to mix in the sugar. Continue to whisking 4 minutes until sugar dissolves. Then mix in the vanilla extract.
3. Place all the ingredients in a food processor or blender, and puree.
4. Pour ingredients into ice cream maker. Let it churn for 25 minutes.
5. Serve immediately.

VANILLA ICE CREAM

Snow Cream Recipe

Ingredients:

- 8 cups clean fresh snow
- 1 (14-ounce) can sweetened condensed milk
- 1 tablespoon vanilla extract

Directions:

1. Mix snow, sweetened condensed milk, and vanilla extract together in a bowl until well mixed.

Rosewater-and-saffron Ice Cream (bastani Irani)?

Ingredients:

- 6 large eggs yolks
- 1 1/2 cups heavy cream
- 1 1/2 cups whole milk
- 3/4 cup sugar
- 1/2 teaspoon kosher salt
- 1/2 teaspoon saffron , finely ground
- 1/4 cup pure rosewater, preferably sadaf brand (see note)
- 1/2 teaspoon pure vanilla extract
- dried roses, for garnish

Directions:

1. Set a medium bowl in a sizable plate of ice water. In another medium bowl, beat the egg yolks until pale, one to two 2 minutes.?
2. In a medium saucepan, whisk the cream with the milk, sugar, salt and saffron. Bring to a simmer over moderate heat, whisking, before sugar is totally dissolved. Very gradually whisk half of the hot cream mixture into the beaten egg yolks in a thin stream, then whisk this mixture back into the saucepan. Cook over moderately low heat, stirring constantly with a wooden spoon, before custard is thick enough to lightly coat the back of the spoon, about ?12 minutes; don't allow it boil.?
3. Strain the custard through a fine-mesh sieve into the bowl set in the ice water. ?Allow custard cool completely, stirring occasionally. Stir in the rosewater and vanilla extract. Press a bit of plastic wrap on the custard and refrigerate until well chilled, at least 4 hours.?

4. Pour the custard base into an ice cream maker and freeze based on the manufacturer's instructions. Transfer the ice cream to a chilled 9-by-4-inch metal loaf pan, cover and freeze until firm, at least ?4 hours.
5. Serve the ice cream in bowls, garnished with dried rose

Roasted Peaches With Mascarpone Ice Cream

Ingredients:

- 4 large eggs yolks
- 3/4 cup plus 2 tablespoons sugar
- 2 cups whole milk
- 1 cup mascarpone (7 ounces)
- 1/2 teaspoon fresh lemon juice
- pinch of salt

Directions:

1. In a sizable bowl, using a handheld mixer, beat the egg yolks with 3/4 cup of the sugar at medium-high speed until fluffy, three minutes. In a saucepan, combine the milk with the remaining 2 tablespoons of the sugar and bring to a simmer. Slowly beat the warm milk in to the egg yolks at low speed. Scrape the custard in to the saucepan. Cook over moderate heat, stirring constantly with a wooden spoon, until thick enough to coat the back of the spoon, about 5 minutes; don't allow the custard boil.
2. Pour the custard right into a bowl set in a larger plate of ice water and whisk in the mascarpone, lemon juice and salt. Let stand until chilled, stirring occasionally, thirty minutes.
3. Pour the custard into an ice cream maker and freeze based on the manufacturer's instructions. Transfer the mascarpone ice cream to an airtight container and freeze until firm, at least 2 hours.
4. In a huge saucepan, combine the white wine, honey, water and sugar and bring to a boil. Boil until reduced by half, about thirty minutes. Add the rosemary sprig and let are a symbol of ten minutes; discard the rosemary.
5. Preheat the oven to 350°. Arrange the peaches within an 8-by-11-inch baking dish. Pour the rosemary syrup at the top and roast the peaches until

tender, 40 minutes, basting and turning the peaches occasionally.

6.   Scoop the mascarpone ice cream into bowls and top with the peach halves. Spoon the warm poaching liquid over the fruit and serve immediately.

Peanut Butter Ice Cream Recipe

Ingredients:
- 4 cups half-and-half cream
- 3 cups non-fat dry milk
- 3 cups milk
- 1 1/2 cups sugar
- 1 1/2 cups peanut butter
- 4 teaspoons vanilla extract

Directions:
1.   Pour the half-and-half, dry milk, and milk into a big saucepan over low heat. Cook until heated, stirring to dissolve the dry milk. Stir in the peanut butter and sugar until smooth and sugar has dissolved. Remove from heat, and stir in the vanilla. Cool mixture, and refrigerate.
2.   Stir the mixture, or merge a blender before pouring into an ice cream maker. Freeze based on the manufacturer's instructions.

Peanut Butter Banana Ice Cream Recipe

Ingredients:
- 4 eaches ripe bananas, cut into 1-inch slices
- 1/4 cup peanut butter

Directions:
1.   Arrange banana slices on a baking sheet and freeze, 8 hours to overnight.
2.   Process frozen bananas in a food processor until evenly chopped; add peanut butter and process until thick and creamy.

Roman's Dairy-free Chocolate-coconut Ice Cream

Ingredients:
- 3 cups unsweetened coconut milk
- 3 tablespoons agave syrup
- 1 1/4 cups sugar

- 2/3 cup unsweetened cocoa powder
- 3 large eggs yolks
- 1 tablespoon pure vanilla extract
- 1/2 cup unsweetened coconut flakes

Directions:
1.   Set a fine-mesh sieve in a big bowl set over a bowl of ice water.
2.   In a huge saucepan, whisk the coconut milk and agave syrup over moderately low heat until warm. In a medium heatproof bowl, whisk the sugar and cocoa powder. Gradually whisk in 1 cup of the warm coconut milk until smooth, then whisk in the egg yolks. Scrape the cocoa paste into the saucepan and whisk until blended. Cook the custard over moderate heat, whisking constantly, for about 6 minutes, until scorching and slightly thickened; don't let it boil. Immediately strain the custard into the prepared bowl and stir in the vanilla. Stir the custard until chilled.
3.   Freeze the custard within an ice cream maker based on the manufacturers' directions. Transfer the ice cream to a big plastic container and freeze until firm, at least 4 hours.
4.   In a little skillet, toast the coconut flakes over low heat until lightly browned, 4 minutes. Transfer to a plate and let cool. Serve the ice cream topped with toasted coconut.

Homemade Mint Chocolate Chip Ice Cream Recipe

Ingredients:
- 2 cups heavy whipping cream
- 1 (14-ounce) can sweetened condensed milk
- 1 cup milk
- 1 teaspoon mint extract
- 1/2 teaspoon vanilla extract
- 1 (12-ounce) bag semisweet chocolate chips

Directions:
1.   Stir heavy cream, sweetened condensed milk, milk, mint extract, vanilla extract, and chocolate chips in a bowl until evenly mixed.
2.   Pour mixture into an ice cream maker and freeze according to manufacturer's directions until softly frozen. Transfer ice cream to a lidded container; cover surface with plastic wrap and seal. For best

results, ice cream should ripen in the freezer for at least 2 hours to overnight.

Caramel-apple Ice Cream

Ingredients:
- 2 tablespoons unsalted butter
- 2 granny smith apples—peeled, quartered and very thinly sliced
- 1 tablespoon sugar
- 1/8 teaspoon cinnamon
- 1/4 cup dulce de leche
- 2 pints vanilla ice cream
- chocolate shavings, for garnish
- crumbled gingersnaps , for garnish

Directions:
1. Melt the butter in a medium skillet. Add the apples and cook over moderate heat, stirring, until softened and browned, about five minutes. Add the sugar, cinnamon and 1/4 cup of water and cook for 2 minutes longer. Stir in the dulce de leche until melted. Scrape the mixture into a bowl and refrigerate until chilled.
2. Fold the apple mixture into softened vanilla ice cream and freeze until firm, about 4 hours. Scoop into bowls and garnish with chocolate shavings and crumbled gingersnaps.

Easy Eggnog Ice Cream Recipe

Ingredients:
- 2 cups eggnog
- 1 cup heavy whipping cream
- 1 cup milk

Directions:
1. Mix the eggnog, whipping cream, and milk together in a bowl, and pour the mixture in to the freezer container of an ice cream maker.
2. Freeze according to manufacturer's directions. Once frozen, spoon the ice cream right into a container, and freeze 2 hours more.

Vanilla Ice Cream Vii Recipe

Ingredients:

- 1 quart heavy cream
- 1 1/4 cups milk
- 1 vanilla bean , split and scraped
- 1 1/4 cups white sugar, divided
- 10 large eggs yolks egg yolks
- 1 tablespoon vanilla extract

Directions:
1. In a heavy saucepan over medium heat, combine cream and milk. Place vanilla bean and scrapings in pot, and sprinkle with half the white sugar. Allow to just come to a boil.
2. Meanwhile, whisk the egg yolks alongside the rest of the sugar and the vanilla extract in a bowl. When the cream is ready, pour a third of it into the egg mixture, and whisk. Pour egg mixture into remaining hot cream and go back to heat until mixture coats the trunk of a metal spoon. Will not boil.
3. Strain custard and chill until cold. Then pour into the canister of an ice cream maker and freeze according to manufacturer's instructions.

Easy Banana Ice Cream Recipe

Ingredients:
- 2 eaches peeled and chopped bananas, frozen
- 1/2 cup skim milk

Directions:
1. Combine frozen bananas and 1/4 cup skim milk in a blender; blend for 30 seconds.
2. Add remaining 1/4 cup milk and blend on high speed until smooth, about 30 seconds more.

Fruited Ice Cream Recipe

Ingredients:
- 2 (14-ounce) cans sweetened condensed milk
- 5 cups milk
- 2 cups heavy cream
- 2 tablespoons vanilla extract
- 1/2 teaspoon salt
- 3 cups chopped strawberries

Directions:
1. Combine condensed milk, milk, cream, vanilla, salt and fruit in freezer canister of ice cream maker.
2. Freeze according to manufacturer's directions.

Strawberry, Lemon And Vanilla Ice Cream Parfait

Ingredients:
- 1 pound strawberries , hulled and quartered
- 1/4 cup granulated sugar
- 1 tablespoon fresh orange juice
- 1/2 teaspoon pure vanilla extract
- 3/4 cup heavy cream
- 1 pint vanilla ice cream
- 4 graham crackers , coarsely crushed
- 1 pint lemon sorbet

Directions:
1. In a food processor, combine the strawberries with the sugar, orange juice and vanilla and pulse before strawberries are coarsely chopped. Let stand before strawberries release some of their juice, about ten minutes. Process the strawberries until smooth.
2. In a medium bowl, utilizing a hand-held mixer, beat the cream at medium speed until soft peaks form.
3. Spoon 2 tablespoons of the strawberry sauce into 4 parfait glasses. Top with a scoop of vanilla ice cream, a sprinkling of the crushed graham crackers, a scoop of the lemon sorbet and another 2 tablespoons of the strawberry sauce. Top the parfaits with a dollop of the whipped cream and finish with a sprinkling of the graham crackers. Serve immediately.

Mermaid Ice Cream

Ingredients:
- 3 cups heavy cream
- 1 14 cans -oz. sweetened condensed milk
- 1 teaspoon pure vanilla extract
- green, blue, and purple food coloring
- sprinkles, for topping (optional)

Directions:
1. In a big bowl utilizing a hand mixer or in the plate of a stand mixer using the whisk attachment, beat heavy cream until medium peaks form.
2. Fold in sweetened condensed milk and vanilla until totally combined, then divide mixture among five bowls. Put in a different color food coloring to each bowl (we used different amounts of green, blue,

and purple) and stir until combined. Layer dollops of the colors in a 9"-x-5" loaf pan until you go out of the mixture.
3. Run a knife through the mixture to swirl the colors three or four 4 times and smooth top.
4. Top with sprinkles (if using) and freeze until firm, 5 hours. Remove from freezer and let soften, 5 to 10 minutes, then scoop and serve.

Peach Ice Cream Recipe

Ingredients:
- 6 large eggs, beaten
- 3 1/2 cups white sugar
- 10 medium (2-1/2" dia) (approx 4 per lb)s fresh peaches , pitted and chopped
- 4 cups heavy cream
- 2 cups half-and-half cream
- 2 teaspoons vanilla extract
- 3/4 teaspoon salt

Directions:
1. In large bowl, mix together eggs and sugar until smooth; puree peaches in blender or food processor and stir 5 cups of puree into egg mixture. Stir in cream, half-and-half, vanilla and salt and mix well.
2. Pour mixture into freezer canister of ice cream maker and freeze according to manufacturer's instructions.

Mocha Espresso Ice Cream Recipe

Ingredients:
- 2 cups heavy whipping cream
- 1 1/2 cups whole milk
- 3/4 cup white sugar
- 1/2 cup brewed espresso , chilled
- 1/4 cup chocolate syrup
- 3/4 cup cocoa roast almonds , chopped
- 4 ounces dark chocolate , chopped

Directions:
1. Mix heavy cream, dairy, sugar, espresso, and chocolate syrup in a bowl until sugar is dissolved. Refrigerate until chilled.
2. Pour the chilled mixture into an ice cream maker and freeze according to manufacturer's directions until it reaches "soft-serve" consistency. Stir in

almonds and chocolates. Serve soft ice cream or transfer ice cream to a one- or two-quart lidded plastic container; cover surface with plastic wrap and seal. For best results, ice cream should ripen in the freezer for at least 2 hours or overnight.

Cookie Butter No-churn Ice Cream

Ingredients:

- 3 cups heavy whipping cream
- 1 14 ounces . can sweetened condensed milk
- 1/4 cup cookie butter, like biscoff
- 2 cups crumbled biscoff cookies, divided

Directions:

1. In a huge bowl, combine heavy whipping cream and condensed milk. Beat with a power mixer on high until stiff peaks form.
2. Slowly fold in cookie butter until well-combined. Sprinkle over 1 cup of crumbled cookies and fold in. Spoon mixture into loaf pan, and freeze for 4 hours or overnight until set.
3. Serve in glasses with remaining crumbled cookie garnish.

Homemade Pumpkin Frozen Yogurt Recipe

Ingredients:

- 2 cups plain whole milk yogurt
- 1 cup whipping cream
- 1 cups raw sugar
- 1 cup pumpkins puree
- 3 tablespoons brandy
- 1 teaspoon vanilla extract
- 1 teaspoon pumpkins pie spice
- Teaspoon sea salt

Directions:

1. Combine the yogurt, cream, sugar, pumpkin puree, brandy, vanilla extract, pumpkin pie spice, and salt in a mixing bowl. Whisk together until the sugar and salt have completely dissolved. Cover, and refrigerate overnight.
2. Pour the chilled mixture into an ice cream maker and freeze according to manufacturer's directions until it reaches "soft-serve" consistency, about 20

minutes. Transfer ice cream to a one- or two-quart lidded container.

3. For best results, ice cream should ripen in the freezer for at least 2 hours or overnight.

The Captain's Mango Ice Cream Recipe

Ingredients:

- 4 eaches mangoes, peeled and cubed
- 2 cups heavy whipping cream
- 3/4 cup packed dark brown sugar
- 1/4 cup light corn syrup
- 4 tablespoons spiced rum
- 1/2 teaspoon kosher salt

Directions:

1. Combine mangoes, cream, brown sugar, and corn syrup in a blender or food processor. Blend on high for 30 seconds.
2. Transfer to an airtight container. Stir in spiced rum and salt. Refrigerate, 8 hours to overnight.
3. Pour mixture into an ice cream maker and freeze according to manufacturer's instructions, about 20 minutes. Transfer to an airtight container and freeze until firm, about 4 hours.

Fast And Easy Creamy Ice Cream Recipe

Ingredients:

- 1 quart half-and-half
- 1 (3.5 ounce) package instant pudding mix, any flavor

Directions:

1. Place the bowl of an ice cream maker in the freezer until completely chilled, at least one hour.
2. Chill half-and-half in the freezer, shaking every ten minutes, until chilled but not frozen, about 30 minutes.
3. Pour chilled half-and-half and pudding mix right into a bowl and mix well with a whisk.
4. Place frozen plate of ice cream maker into the ice cream maker; add the stirring component and lid. Turn on the machine so the bowl is rotating. Pour pudding mixture into the machine through the hole in the lid.

5. Allow ice cream to process in the ice cream maker until desired consistency is reached, about 30 minutes.

Easy Ice Cream In A Bag Recipe

Ingredients:
- 1/4 cup milk
- 1/4 cup half-and-half
- 1 tablespoon white sugar
- 1/4 teaspoon vanilla extract
- 1 cup ice cubes, or as needed
- 3 tablespoons ice cream rock salt

Directions:
1. Combine milk, half-and-half, sugar, and vanilla extract in a pint-size resealable plastic bag; seal tightly.
2. Put a scoop of ice, 3 tablespoons ice cream rock salt, and the bag containing the milk-cream mixture right into a gallon-size resealable plastic bag; seal tightly.
3. Rock the bag backwards and forwards (usually do not shake) until contents thicken into ice cream, about 10 minutes. Wipe salt from the very best of the pint-size bag before opening to prevent salt from getting into the ice cream.

No-churn Cake Batter Ice Cream Recipe

Ingredients:
- 2 cups heavy whipping cream
- 1 (14-ounce) can sweetened condensed milk
- 1 1/4 cups cake mix with candy bits (such as pills bury funfetti), or more to taste

Directions:
1. Beat cream with an electric mixer in a sizable bowl until stiff peaks form.
2. Stir condensed milk and cake mix together in another bowl. Fold cake mix mixture into whipped cream. Pour mixture into a freezer-safe container, cover the container, and freeze until ice cream is defined, 6 hours to overnight.

Keto No-churn Strawberry Ice Cream Recipe

Ingredients:
- 1 cup heavy whipping cream
- 1/3 cup chopped strawberries
- 2 tablespoons low-calorie natural sweetener (such as swerve)
- 1 tablespoon vodka
- 1 teaspoon vanilla extract
- 1/4 teaspoon xanthan gum
- 1 pinch salt

Directions:
1. Combine heavy cream, strawberries, sweetener, vodka, vanilla extract, xanthan gum, and salt in a wide-mouth pint-size jar.
2. Using an immersion blender and an along motion, blend cream mixture for 60 to 75 seconds, or until thickened and soft peaks have formed.
3. Cover jar and freeze, stirring every 30 to 40 minutes, until ice cream reaches your ideal consistency, 3 to 4 hours.

Chunky Banana Nut Chip Ice Cream Recipe

Ingredients:
- 4 medium (7" to 7-7/8" long)s bananas, broken into chunks
- 1 tablespoon lemon juice
- 1 teaspoon vanilla extract
- 1 cup white sugar
- 1 1/3 cups heavy cream , chilled
- 2/3 cup cold milk
- 1/2 cup chopped toasted walnuts
- 1/2 cup miniature semisweet chocolate chips

Directions:
1. In a blender or food processor, combine bananas, lemon juice, vanilla, sugar, cream and milk. Puree until smooth. Transfer mixture to the freezer canister of an ice cream maker and freeze according to manufacturer's instructions.
2. When ice cream starts to stiffen, add walnuts and chocolate chips.

Easy Banana Ice Cream With Milk Chocolate Chunks

Ingredients:

- 3 ripe bananas
- 1 1/4 cups whole milk
- 1/3 cup sugar
- 1 teaspoon pure vanilla extract
- 1/8 teaspoon salt
- 1/2 cup heavy cream
- 3 ounces milk chocolate (preferably with nibs), chopped into 1/4-inch chunks

Directions:

1. In a blender, puree the bananas with the milk, sugar, vanilla, and salt until smooth. Transfer to a bowl and stir in a heavy cream and milk chocolate.
2. Pour the banana custard into an ice cream maker and freeze based on the manufacturer's instructions. Transfer the ice cream to an airtight container and freeze until firm, at least 4 hours. Let stand at room temperature for ten minutes before serving.

Guinness Ice Cream Recipe

Ingredients:

- 2 cups heavy whipping cream
- 1 1/2 cups whole milk
- 1 cup white sugar
- 1 vanilla bean
- 6 large eggs yolks egg yolks, beaten
- 1 (12 fluid ounce) can or bottle irish stout beer (such as guinness)

Directions:

1. Combine cream, milk, and sugar in a saucepan over medium heat. Stir until sugar has dissolved, about five minutes.
2. Split the vanilla bean lengthwise with a sharp knife and scrape seeds into cream mixture. Place bean pod into mixture and bring to a boil. Remove from heat and discard vanilla bean pod.
3. Place egg yolks in a bowl. Gradually whisk in 1 cup hot cream mixture.
4. Whisk the egg yolk mixture back again to the saucepan and place over medium heat. Whisk constantly until slightly thickened, about 2-3 3

minutes. Mixture should coat the trunk of a spoon. Don't let the mixture boil.

5. Transfer cream mixture to a bowl and chill until cold, at least 2 hours to overnight.
6. Simmer Irish stout beer in a saucepan over low heat until reduced to 2/3 cup, in regards to a quarter-hour. Chill the stout beer syrup at least 2 hours to overnight.
7. Whisk together chilled cream mixture and beer syrup; pour into an ice cream maker and freeze according to manufacturer's directions.
8. When machine has finished, pack ice cream right into a airtight container and store in freezer.

Orange-pineapple Ice Recipe

Ingredients:

- 1 (14-ounce) can sweetened condensed milk
- 1 (8-ounce) can crushed pineapple
- 1 gallon orange soda

Directions:

1. Combine condensed milk, pineapple and orange soda in freezer canister of ice cream maker. Freeze according to manufacturer's directions.

Mudslide No-churn Ice Cream

Ingredients:

- 2 cups heavy cream
- 1 ounce 14.5- can sweetened condensed milk
- 1 cup chopped chocolate
- 1/4 cup hot fudge sauce , plus more for serving
- 2 tablespoons kahlua
- 2 tablespoons baileys irish cream

Directions:

1. In a stand mixer fitted with a whisk attachment, beat heavy cream until stiff peaks form, 5 minutes. Fold in sweetened condensed milk until fully combined, then fold in chocolate, fudge sauce, Kahlua, and Baileys.
2. Transfer mixture to a 9-x-5" loaf pan and add one more chocolate swirl on top. Freeze 5 hours. When ready to serve, let soften 10 minutes. Serve with warm hot fudge.

Peanut Butter Cup Ice Cream Recipe

Ingredients:
- 1/4 cup sugar
- 3 large eggs
- 1 cup whole milk
- 3/4 cup peanut butter
- 3/4 cup sweetened condensed milk
- 1/2 cup half-and-half cream
- 2 teaspoons vanilla extract
- 12 eaches miniature peanut butter cups, chopped

Directions:
1. In a medium bowl, beat the sugar and eggs with an electric mixer until thick, about three minutes. Set aside. Pour milk into a small saucepan, and bring to a simmer over low heat. Gradually drizzle the hot milk into the eggs while whisking vigorously. Then pour the whole mixture into the saucepan. Cook over low heat, stirring constantly, until thick enough to coat the back of a metal spoon. Usually do not boil.
2. Remove from heat, and whisk in peanut butter. Allow to cool slightly, then whisk in the sweetened condensed milk, half-and-half and vanilla. Cover and refrigerate until chilled.
3. Pour the mixture into an ice cream maker, and freeze based on the manufacturer's instructions. Fold in peanut butter cups when mixture continues to be soft, then transfer to a container, and freeze until solid.

Mint Mojito Coffee Ice Cream Recipe

Ingredients:
- 2 cups whole milk
- 1/3 cup coarsely ground coffee beans
- 3/4 cup brown sugar, divided
- 1 bunch fresh mint leaves, crushed
- 6 large eggs yolks large egg yolks
- 1 cup heavy whipping cream
- 1/3 cup white rum
- 1/3 cup chopped chocolate

Directions:
1. Heat milk, ground coffee, 1/4 cup brown sugar, and mint in a saucepan over low heat until warmed through, 7 to ten minutes.

2. Whisk egg yolks and remaining 1/2 cup brown sugar in a bowl; slowly whisk in about 1 cup hot milk mixture. Pour egg yolk mixture into saucepan and continue steadily to heat until custard is thickened, about five minutes.
3. Line a sieve with cheesecloth and strain custard into a large bowl; discard solids. Whisk heavy cream into custard. Cover and refrigerate until chilled, 4 to 5 hours.
4. Stir rum and chocolate into chilled custard and pour into an ice cream maker. Freeze according to manufacturer's directions.

Smooth Raspberry Ice Cream Recipe

Ingredients:
- 4 cups fresh raspberries
- 2 large eggs
- 1 1/3 cups white sugar
- 1 1/2 cups half-and-half
- 1 cup heavy whipping cream
- 1/4 cup light corn syrup
- 1 tablespoon lemon juice

Directions:
1. Puree raspberries in a blender or food processor; pour mixture through a strainer to eliminate seeds.
2. Beat eggs and sugar together in a bowl until smooth. Stir raspberry puree, half-and-half, cream, corn syrup, and lemon juice into the egg-sugar mixture.
3. Transfer raspberry cream mixture to the ice cream maker. Freeze according to the manufacturer's instructions.

Vegan Blueberry Coconut Ice Cream Recipe

Ingredients:
- 2 tablespoons roasted flax seeds
- 2 (15-ounce) cans full-fat coconut milk , chilled
- 2 cups blueberries
- 1 tablespoon lemon juice
- 1 teaspoon vanilla extract
- 1 teaspoon coconut oils
- 1 teaspoon stevia powder

- 1/2 teaspoon xanthan gum, or more as desired
- 1/4 teaspoon himalayan black salt

Directions:

1. Pulse flax seeds in a coffee grinder until finely ground.
2. Combine 1 can coconut milk, blueberries, and lemon juice in a blender; puree until blueberry skins breakdown completely. Add ground flax seeds, remaining coconut milk, vanilla extract, coconut oil, stevia, xanthan gum, and salt; puree until very smooth.
3. Transfer blender container to the freezer to chill mixture briefly, about 15 minutes
4. Pour mixture into an ice cream maker and churn according to manufacturer's instructions, about 20 minutes. Transfer to a lidded container before serving.

Tropical Avocado Ice Cream

Ingredients:

- 4 avocados , peeled and pitted
- 1 cup lime juice (about 4 juicy limes)
- zest of 2 lime
- 1 cup maple syrup
- 2 cans coconut cream
- 2 teaspoons vanilla extract
- 2 tablespoons coconut oils
- 1/2 teaspoon kosher salt
- 1/2 lime, thinly sliced into quarters, for garnish

Directions:

1. Combine all ingredients, except lime slices, in a blender. Blend on high until smooth.
2. Pour into loaf pan and garnish with lime slices. Freeze until firm, at least 3 hours or overnight.

Lina And Jens' Delicious Vegan Chocolate Ice Cream Recipe

Ingredients:

- 7 ounces dark chocolate , chopped
- 1 1/4 cups aquafaba
- 1/2 teaspoon xanthan gum
- 1/2 cup confectioners' sugar
- 2 teaspoons vanilla sugar

Directions:

1. Melt chocolate in top of a double boiler over simmering water, stirring frequently and scraping down the sides with a rubber spatula in order to avoid scorching. Let cool slightly, about ten minutes.
2. Pour aquafaba in to the plate of a stand mixer fitted with a whisk attachment. Beat on high speed until fluffy and quadrupled in volume, about 1 minute. Add xanthan gum and beat for 30 seconds. Add confectioners' sugar and vanilla sugar; continue beating until foam is firm and glossy, about 2 minutes more.
3. Fold melted chocolate gently into whipped foam until thoroughly incorporated. Transfer to a lidded container.
4. Freeze until firm, 8 hours to overnight.

Condensed-milk Ice Cream With Black Sesame Polvoron?

Ingredients:

- 2 cups heavy cream
- 1 (14-ounce) can sweetened condensed milk
- 1/4 cup brown rice flour
- 1/2 cup black sesame seeds
- 1/2 cup powdered milk
- 1/4 cup granulated sugar
- 1/4 cup unsalted butter, melted

Directions:

1. Place cream in a huge chilled bowl; beat with a power mixer until stiff peaks form, 2 to 3 three minutes. Gently fold in condensed milk until fully incorporated (do not overmix). Cover bowl with plastic wrap to ensure that plastic rests on surface of mixture. Freeze until firm, 8 to 10 hours.
2. Preheat oven to 325°F. Line a rimmed baking sheet with parchment paper. Spread rice flour in a thin layer on prepared baking sheet. Toast in preheated oven until flour smells nutty and is sandy in color, 12 to 14 minutes. Reserve. On a second parchment-lined rimmed baking sheet, spread sesame seeds in a thin, even layer, and toast until fragrant, six to eight 8 minutes. Let stand until cool.?
3. Place 1/3 cup toasted sesame seeds in the bowl of a food processor. Pulse until seeds are coarsely ground, about 8 times.?

4. Sift powdered milk, sugar, and toasted rice flour into a big bowl. Add ground sesame seeds and remaining toasted sesame seeds to bowl. Gently stir in melted butter. Let cool; transfer to an airtight container.?

5. To serve, spoon 3 small scoops of ice cream into a bowl, and sprinkle liberally with sesame mixture.

Mint-chip Coconut Milk Ice Cream Recipe

Ingredients:

- 24 fluid ounces canned coconut milk
- 1/3 cup agave syrup, or to taste
- 1 teaspoon peppermint extract, or to taste
- 3 ounces dark chocolate , chopped into small pieces

Directions:

1. Chill all the ingredients prior to preparing to quicken the freezing process

2. Blend coconut milk in a blender until smooth and evenly mixed; add agave syrup and peppermint extract and blend until smooth.

3. Transfer coconut milk mixture to an ice cream maker and follow manufacturer's instructions for ice cream, adding chocolate pieces when indicated. Freeze for 2 hours before serving.

Six Threes Ice Cream Recipe

Ingredients:

- 3 cups sugar
- 3 cups cream
- 3 cups milk
- 3 medium (7" to 7-7/8" long)s bananas, mashed
- 3 fruit, (2-5/8" dia, sphere)s oranges , juiced
- 3 fruit, without seeds lemons, juiced

Directions:

1. In a huge bowl, whisk together sugar and cream until sugar is dissolved. Mix in the milk, mashed bananas, and fruit drinks.

2. Pour mixture into ice cream maker. Freeze according to manufacturer's directions, about 45 minutes.

Cinnamon Ice Cream Ii Recipe

Ingredients:

- 3/4 cup heavy cream
- 2 tablespoons sour cream
- 6 large eggs
- 2/3 cup sugar
- 2 cups milk
- 1 tablespoon ground cinnamon
- 1 teaspoon vanilla extract

Directions:

1. In a medium bowl, stir together the heavy cream and sour cream. Reserve in a warm place for approximately an hour to thicken.

2. In another bowl, beat eggs with sugar using an electric mixer until pale. Stir in the milk and cinnamon, and transfer to a saucepan. Bring to a simmer over medium-low heat. Cook, stirring constantly, until thick enough to coat the trunk of a metal spoon. Stir in the vanilla, and remove from the heat. Reserve to cool.

3. When the custard has cooled, stir in the sour cream mixture. Freeze in an ice cream maker based on the manufacturer's instructions.

Vanilla Ice Cream Ix Recipe

Ingredients:

- 4 large eggs
- 2 1/2 cups white sugar
- 2 cups heavy cream
- 2 cups evaporated milk
- 5 cups whole milk
- 2 1/4 teaspoons vanilla extract
- 2 1/4 teaspoons lemon extract
- 1/2 teaspoon salt

Directions:

1. In a mixing bowl, beat eggs and sugar until stiff. Stir in cream, evaporated milk, dairy, vanilla, lemon extract and salt until well combined.

2. Pour into the freezer canister of an ice cream maker and freeze according to manufacturer's instructions.

Ice Cream Cones

Ingredients:
- 1 large sheet heavy-duty aluminum foil (20x12 inch)
- 2 large eggs whites large egg whites, room temperature
- 1/2 cup white sugar
- 1/2 cup packed all-purpose flour , plus more if needed
- 2 tablespoons whole milk
- 2 tablespoons melted butter
- 1 tablespoon cold water, or as needed
- 1/4 teaspoon vanilla extract
- 1 teaspoon kosher salt

Directions:
1. Preheat oven to 400 degrees F (200 degrees C). Line a rimmed baking sheet with a silicone baking mat.
2. Fold aluminum foil in half and bunch it up to create a solid cone form with a pointy end and a wider end about how big is an ice cream cone. This will be utilized to shape the cones if they come out of the oven.
3. Whisk egg whites and sugar together in a mixing bowl until mixture is smooth and shiny, about 2 minutes. Add flour, milk, melted butter, water, vanilla, and salt. Whisk together until thoroughly combined.
4. Ladle about one to two 2 tablespoons batter on 1 side of silicone mat on prepared baking sheet. Gently swirl the batter with the trunk of the ladle outwards to make a fairly thin flat circle 5 or 6 inches in diameter. If necessary, you may use a pastry brush to even the thickness. If batter seems too thin, add a bit more flour. If too thick, more water. Bake in batches, 2 per batch.
5. Bake in preheated oven until edges are browned around the outside few inches, about 8 minutes.
6. Gently loosen among the circles. While still hot, place the aluminum foil cone mold using one end and roll the circle right into a cone shape, pressing together the pointed bottom to seal it. Put on a cooking rack seam side down. You may need to put the pan back the oven for one minute to heat the next circle; they must be hot to wrap around the mold. Repeat for the rest of the cones.

Olive Oil Ice Cream

Ingredients:
- 1/2 cup granulated sugar
- 2 tablespoons nonfat powdered milk
- 1/4 teaspoon xanthan gum
- 1 1/3 cups whole milk
- 2 tablespoons light corn syrup
- 1 1/3 cups heavy cream
- 1/4 cup grassy extra-virgin olive oils (such as red ridge farm durant arbequina), plus more for garnish
- 1/2 teaspoon kosher salt
- flaky sea salt (such as maldon)

Directions:
1. Stir together sugar, powdered milk, and xanthan gum in a little bowl. Whisk together milk and corn syrup in a medium saucepan. Add sugar mixture, and whisk until smooth. Heat mixture over medium, whisking often, until sugar has fully dissolved, three to four 4 minutes. (Usually do not simmer.) Remove from heat, and whisk in cream. Cover and chill at least 6 hours. For better still texture and flavor, chill mixture up to 24 hours. Base can be stored within an airtight container in freezer for three months; thaw completely before using.
2. Whisk together chilled base, olive oil, and kosher salt until well combined. (There it's still little droplets of oil on the surface.) Pour mixture into freezer bowl of a 11/2-quart electric ice cream maker and proceed according to manufacturer's directions until ice cream has the texture of soft-serve, about 35 minutes. (Instructions and times may vary.)
3. Quickly transfer ice cream to a freezer-safe container; press parchment paper directly onto surface. Cover container, and freeze until firm, at least 6 hours. Ice cream can be kept in freezer up to three months. To serve, garnish with olive oil and flaky sea salt.

Frozen Vanilla Custard

Ingredients:
- 5 large eggs yolks
- 2/3 cup white sugar
- 1 pinch salt

- 1 cup whole milk
- 2 cups heavy cream
- 2 1/2 teaspoons pure vanilla extract

Directions:

1. Whisk egg yolks, sugar, and salt together until mixture changes from dark golden to pale yellow becomes fluffy.
2. Heat milk and cream in much saucepan over medium heat. Stir occasionally to avoid sticking to underneath. Cook just until mixture starts to simmer when little bubbles begin to appear on the top, 5 to 8 minutes. Remove from heat.
3. Whisk a ladleful of milk-cream mixture into the egg yolk mixture. Add another ladleful and whisk thoroughly before adding the next (this could keep the eggs from cooking). Gradually add the rest of the milk-cream mixture and whisk thoroughly. Whisk in vanilla. Cool completely (you can place the bowl in a more substantial bowl with ice water to cool it faster).
4. Pour cooled mixture right into a pitcher; cover. Refrigerate until ice cold or overnight.
5. Pour custard mixture into ice cream maker and process (according to manufacturer's instructions) until custard reaches the consistency of soft ice cream, about 20 minutes. Quickly transfer to a plastic container.
6. Place a bit of plastic wrap over the top of custard. Cover container and freeze until custard is firm enough to scoop, at least 3 hours.

Salted Pecan-maple Ice Cream Recipe

Ingredients:

- 1/2 cup coarsely chopped pecans
- 2 tablespoons white sugar
- 1/2 teaspoon sea salt , or to taste
- 3/4 cup white sugar
- 1/4 cup real maple syrup
- 2 large eggs
- 1 teaspoon vanilla extract
- 1 drop maple-flavored extract, or to taste
- 3 cups half-and-half
- 1 pinch coarse sea salt , or to taste

Directions:

1. Place pecans right into a heavy saucepan over medium heat and toast the nuts, stirring constantly, until fragrant, one to two 2 minutes.
2. Sprinkle 2 tablespoons sugar over pecans and stir constantly before sugar melts to a light brown syrup and coats the pecans. Immediately pull the pan off the heat; sprinkle with 1/2 teaspoon sea salt.
3. Turn hot pecans out onto a bit of parchment paper and cool thoroughly; break apart any large clumps. Set candied pecans aside.
4. Whisk 3/4 cup sugar, maple syrup, eggs, vanilla extract, and maple flavoring in a sizable bowl until smooth. Slowly whisk in half-and-half.
5. Pour mixture into an ice cream maker and freeze according to manufacturer's instructions. Mix the candied pecans in to the softly-frozen ice cream. Sprinkle servings with a pinch of coarsely ground sea salt.

Guinness Ice Cream With Chocolate-covered Pretzels

Ingredients:

- 2 cups guinness (16 ounces)
- 2 cups heavy cream
- 1 3/4 cups whole milk
- 15 large eggs yolks
- 1 cup granulated sugar
- chocolate-covered pretzels , for serving

Directions:

1. In a sizable saucepan, combine the Guinness with the cream and milk and bring to a simmer over moderately high temperature. In a huge bowl, whisk the egg yolks with the sugar. Gradually add the hot Guinness cream to the yolks, whisking constantly until well blended.
2. Pour the mixture in to the saucepan and cook over moderate heat, stirring constantly until it coats the trunk of a spoon, about 6 minutes; don't let it boil. Pour the custard into a medium bowl set in a large bowl filled up with ice water. Let stand before custard is cold, stirring occasionally, about thirty minutes.
3. Pour the custard into an ice cream maker and freeze based on the manufacturer's instructions (this may have to be done in 2 batches).

4. Pack the ice cream into an airtight container and freeze until firm, about 4 hours.

5. Spoon the ice cream into bowls and top with some Chocolate-Covered Pretzels. Serve simultaneously.

Tropical Ice Cream Recipe

Ingredients:

- 2 cups heavy cream
- 1 1/3 cups 2% low-fat milk
- 2/3 cup pineapple and orange juice blend
- 3/4 cup sugar
- 1/3 cup flaked sweetened coconut
- 1/3 cup walnut pieces
- 1 large banana, sliced

Directions:

1. Whisk together cream, milk, pineapple-orange juice, and sugar until the sugar has dissolved. Pour into an ice cream maker and freeze according to manufacturer's instructions.

2. Five minutes prior to the ice cream is performed, add the coconut and walnut pieces. Two minutes prior to the ice cream is performed, add the sliced banana.

Coffee And Doughnuts Ice Cream Recipe

Ingredients:

- 3 doughnut (3-3/4" dia)s day-old glazed doughnuts, cut into 8 pieces
- 1 cup cold, strong, brewed coffee
- 1/2 cup sugar
- 2 cups heavy cream
- 1 (14-ounce) can sweetened condensed milk
- 1/2 cup milk
- 1 teaspoon vanilla extract

Directions:

1. Place the doughnut pieces within a layer in the bottom of a shallow dish. Pour just enough of the coffee over the doughnuts so the liquid is totally absorbed by the doughnuts. Put the dish in the freezer.

2. Mix the remaining coffee with the sugar, cream, sweetened condensed milk, milk, and vanilla in a bowl; stir.

3. Pour the mixture into an ice cream maker and freeze according to manufacturer's directions before ice cream cycle is completed. Fold the frozen doughnuts in to the mixture; transfer ice cream to a one- or two-quart lidded plastic container; cover surface with plastic wrap and seal. Ripen in the freezer for at least 12 hours.

Snow Ice Cream

Ingredients:

- 1 cup (8 oz.) sweetened condensed milk
- 1/3 cup sugar
- 1 teaspoon pure vanilla extract
- 4 cups snow
- sprinkles, for garnish if desired

Directions:

1. In a medium bowl, combine sweetened condensed milk, sugar and vanilla. Whisk until smooth. In a large bowl, pour condensed milk mixture over snow.

2. Stir to combine. Freeze 30 minutes to 1 hour or until almost solid. Scoop into bowls and serve. Garnish with sprinkles if desired.

Pumpkin Ice Cream

Ingredients:

- 1 15 cans 1 (15-oz.) pumpkins puree
- 2 cups whole milk
- 2 cups heavy cream
- 1 cup packed brown sugar
- 6 large eggs yolks
- 1 teaspoon pure vanilla extract
- 1 teaspoon cinnamon
- 1/2 teaspoon ginger
- 1/2 teaspoon nutmeg
- 1/4 teaspoon kosher salt

Directions:

1. The day before you intend to churn, freeze the plate of your ice cream maker. As your ice cream base will have to chill as well, we suggest which makes it the night time before, too.

2. In a medium saucepan over medium heat, whisk together pumpkin puree, milk, and cream. When mixture starts to boil, remove from heat and set aside.

In a sizable bowl, whisk brown sugar and egg yolks until pale and thick ribbons form, three to four 4 minutes. (You might use a hand mixer.) Whisking constantly, gradually add about 50 % of hot pumpkin mixture to eggs, one ladle at a time, to warm mixture through.

3.	Pour mixture back to saucepan with remaining pumpkin mixture. Return pan over low heat and cook, stirring frequently with a wooden spoon, until mixture thickens, making sure the mixture never comes up to a simmer, about 4 to five minutes. To check on if the mixture is done, coat the trunk of your wooden spoon with the mixture and swipe your finger through the mixture.

4.	If your finger leaves a clean line, your mixture is good to go-this will be at around 170°, if you are using a candy thermometer.

5.	When the custard is adequately thickened, stir in vanilla and spices. Strain into a sizable bowl and place over an ice bath. Let cool to room temperature, then cover and chill at least 3 hours, up to overnight. Whenever your custard is chilled as well as your ice cream maker bowl is frozen, churn ice cream according to manufacturer's instructions, about a quarter-hour, scraping sides occasionally.

6.	When ice cream is soft-serve consistency, transfer to another container and freeze until hardened, 2-3 3 hours, up to overnight.

Pecan Caramel Ice Cream Recipe

Ingredients:
- 1 cup caramel ice cream topping
- 3 1/2 cups milk
- 1 (14-ounce) can sweetened condensed milk (such as eagle brand®)
- 1 (3.5 ounce) package instant vanilla pudding mix
- 1 teaspoon vanilla extract
- 1/2 teaspoon salt
- 1 1/2 cups coarsely chopped pecans, or more to taste

Directions:
1.	Place caramel ice cream topping right into a microwave-safe container and heat in microwave until slightly warmed and softened, 10 to 30 seconds.

2.	Whisk caramel topping, milk, sweetened condensed milk, instant vanilla pudding mix, vanilla extract and salt in a huge mixing bowl until pudding mix has dissolved and batter is smooth.

3.	Cover bowl and chill batter thoroughly, at least 6 hours to overnight.

4.	Pour chilled batter into an ice cream maker and freeze according to manufacturer's instructions; stir pecans into soft ice cream at end of freezing time.

5.	Serve soft if desired. If a harder ice cream is recommended, pack pecan ice cream right into a lidded container and freeze to desired consistency

Ice Cream Base Recipe

Ingredients:
- 1 cup heavy cream
- 3 cups half-and-half cream
- 8 large eggs yolks egg yolks
- 1 cup white sugar
- 1 teaspoon salt

Directions:
1.	Pour the heavy cream and half-and-half cream heavy saucepan, place over medium-low heat, and heat until barely simmering, stirring frequently. Turn down to low.

2.	Whisk together the egg yolks, sugar, and salt in bowl until thoroughly combined.

3.	Slowly pour about 1/2 cup of hot cream mixture egg yolk mixture|is better, whisking constantly. Repeat more, whisking thoroughly before adding each additional 1/2 cup of hot cream to the egg yolk mixture. Pour the egg yolk mixture the saucepan with hot cream, and whisk constantly over medium-low heat mixture thickens coat of a spoon, 5 to 8 minutes. mixture boil.

4.	Pour the ice cream base bowl to cool 20 minutes; place in refrigerator and chill overnight. , pour into an ice cream maker, and freeze manufacturer's directions. ice cream, pack covered container, and freeze for 2 hours or overnight before serving.

Simple Mint Chocolate Chip Strawberry Ice Cream Recipe

Ingredients:

- 2 cups whipping cream heavy whipping cream
- 1 cup milk whole milk
- 1/2 cup sugar white sugar
- 1/2 teaspoon peppermint extract pure peppermint extract
- 2 ounces chocolate dark chocolate finely chopped
- 6 strawberries medium (1-1/4" dia)s fresh strawberries diced

Directions:

1. Mix heavy cream, whole milk, sugar, and peppermint extract in a bowl.

2. Pour mixture into an ice cream maker and freeze until slightly thickened, 25 to 30 minutes (time varies according to ice cream maker specifications). Stir chocolate and strawberries into ice cream mixture; allow to combine until thickened, 3 to 5 5 more minutes.

Tart Lemon Ice Cream Recipe

Ingredients:

- 1 large lemon, juiced and zested
- 1 cup white sugar
- 1 cup milk
- 1 cup heavy cream , chilled

Directions:

1. Combine the lemon zest and sugar in the container of a food processor. Blend before zest is very fine. In a medium bowl, stir together the sugar and milk until sugar has dissolved, then stir in the lemon juice. In another bowl, whip the heavy cream until stiff however, not grainy. Gently fold the whipped cream in to the lemon mixture until evenly blended.

2. Pour the mixture right into a 9x5 inch loaf pan, and cover with plastic wrap. Freeze for 3 hours, or until firm.

Key Lime Ice Cream Recipe

Ingredients:

- 2 eggs large egg
- 1 <small>1/4</small> cups sugar white sugar
- 4 eggs large egg yolks egg yolks
- 1 tablespoon lemon zest lemon zest

- 2 <small>1/4</small> cups cream half-and-half cream
- 3/4 cup lime juice lime juice

Directions:

1. hisk together the eggs, egg yolks, sugar, lime juice, and lemon zest in a saucepan over medium heat until well-blended. Continuously stir the egg mixture with a wooden spoon until thickened, 7 to 8 minutes. The mixture ought to be thick enough to coat the trunk of the spoon. Remove from heat, and stir in the half and half until smooth. Strain the mixture through a fine sieve set over a clean bowl. Cover and chill the mixture in the refrigerator, stirring occasionally, until cool, about 1 hour.

2. Pour the chilled mixture into an ice cream maker and freeze according to manufacturer's directions until it reaches "soft-serve" consistency. Transfer ice cream to a one- or two-quart lidded plastic container; cover surface with plastic wrap and seal. For best results, ice cream should ripen in the freezer for at least 2 hours or overnight.

Chocolate Snow Ice Cream Recipe

Ingredients:

- 2 cups milk
- 1 cup confectioners' sugar
- 1 tablespoon vanilla extract
- 1/4 cup unsweetened cocoa powder
- 1 teaspoon powdered instant coffee
- 1 gallon clean fresh snow

Directions:

1. In a bowl, whisk together the milk, confectioners' sugar, vanilla extract, cocoa powder, and instant coffee until the sugar has dissolved and the mixture is smooth.

2. Place the snow into a huge bowl, and pour the chocolate mixture over the snow. With a huge spoon, stir until the snow ice cream is thoroughly combined. Serve immediately.

Truly Key Lime Pie Ice Cream Recipe

Ingredients:

- 1 (12 fluid ounce) can evaporated milk
- 1 (14-ounce) can sweetened condensed milk

- 2 cups milk
- 2/3 cup heavy cream
- 2 large eggs yolks egg yolks, beaten
- 1 cup white sugar
- 1 cup lime juice
- 2 teaspoons lemon extract
- 1 (3-ounce) package lime flavored jell-o mixes
- 6 large rectangular piece or 2 squares or 4 small rectangular pieces whole graham crackers

Directions:

1. In a saucepan over low heat, combine the evaporated milk, sweetened condensed milk, milk, and heavy cream. Cook until warm, whisking frequently. Once the mixture is hot to touch, whisk in the gelatin mix and sugar, stirring constantly until sugar and gelatin are completely dissolved. Whisk in the egg yolks, and remove from the heat. Stir in the lime juice and lemon extract.

2. Pour the mixture into an ice cream maker, and freeze based on the manufacturer's instructions. This recipe takes a little longer to create than the usual ice cream.

3. After the ice cream is thick, open the canister, and place large bits of graham cracker evenly on each side. They will break right into smaller pieces as the device churns. Mix for about 5 more minutes. Transfer to a freezer container, seal, and freeze until solid. I like to use 1 gallon resealable freezer bags.

Vanilla Ice Cream Recipe

Ingredients:

- 8 cups milk
- 2 cups white sugar
- 1 tablespoon vanilla extract

Directions:

1. Combine milk, sugar and vanilla in freezer canister of ice cream maker.

2. Freeze according to manufacturer's instructions.

Five Minute Ice Cream

Ingredients:

- 1 (10-ounce) package frozen sliced strawberries
- 1/2 cup sugar
- 2/3 cup heavy cream

Directions:

1. Combine the frozen strawberries and sugar in a food processor or blender.

2. Process until the fruit is roughly chopped. With the processor running, slowly pour in the heavy cream until fully incorporated. Serve immediately or freeze for up to one week.

Dark Brownie Fudge Ice Cream Recipe

Ingredients:

- 1 cup heavy whipping cream
- 3/4 cup whole milk
- 1/4 teaspoon ground espresso beans
- 1/3 cup semi-sweet chocolate chips
- 1 cup packed dark brown sugar
- 2 tablespoons dutch dark cocoa powder
- 1/4 cup unsalted butter
- 1 tablespoon vanilla extract

Directions:

1. Combine whipping cream and milk in a little saucepan over medium heat. Cook for 2 minutes. Stir in ground espresso. Gently add chocolate chips and stir continuously until chocolate melts and is fully blended with the cream mixture, making sure nothing sticks to underneath of the pan.

2. Stir in brown sugar until dissolved, reducing heat to low when the mixture starts to boil. Mix in cocoa powder until incorporated. Add butter; stir until melted. Stir in vanilla extract. Continue stirring over low heat until mixture is dark brown and smooth.

3. Pass the mixture through an excellent strainer to remove espresso granules, then pour into an ice cream maker and freeze according to manufacturer's instructions, about 20 minutes. Transfer to an airtight container and freeze until firm, about 4 hours.

Creamy Pomegranate Ice Cream Recipe

Ingredients:

- 1 cup heavy cream
- 1 cup white sugar
- 1 cup pomegranate juice
- 1 teaspoon vanilla extract
- 1 pinch salt

Directions:

1. The first step 1 Stir together the heavy cream and sugar. Stir in the pomegranate juice, vanilla extract, and salt.
2. Add the mixture to an ice cream maker and freeze predicated on the manufacturer's directions.

Unicorn Ice Cream

Ingredients:

- 3 cups heavy cream
- 1 11 cans -oz. sweetened condensed milk
- 1 teaspoon pure vanilla extract
- 2 drops each assorted food coloring (pink, purple, green, blue, yellow)
- sprinkles, for topping (optional)

Directions:

1. In a huge bowl using a hand mixer or in the bowl of a stand mixer using the whisk attachment, whisk heavy cream until medium peaks form.
2. Fold in sweetened condensed milk and vanilla until totally combined, then divide mixture among 5 bowls. Put in a different color food coloring to each bowl (we used pink, purple, green, blue and yellow) and stir until combined. Layer dollops of the colors in a 9"-x-5" loaf pan until you go out of the mixture.
3. Smooth the very best and run a knife through the mixture to swirl the colors (don't overmix if not the colors can be muddy; 4 to 5 swirls ought to be plenty). Top with sprinkles (if using) and freeze until firm, 5 hours. Remove from freezer and let soften, 5 to ten minutes, then scoop and serve.

Instant Strawberry Ice Cream Recipe

Ingredients:

- 24 ounces frozen sweetened strawberries , cut into large chunks
- 1/2 cup sugar, plus
- 1 tablespoon sugar
- 1 1/2 cups heavy cream

Directions:

1. Place berries in blender. Whisk sugar into cream. With blender going, slowly add cream through opening in lid, stopping to stir the mixture three or four 4 times therefore the ice cream is smooth, with small items of berries.
2. Transfer to shallow pan and freeze to a scoopable texture, about 2 hours. Garnish with fresh strawberries, if you want.

Ice Cream Salad Recipe

Ingredients:

- 1/2 (8-ounce) package reduced-fat cream cheese , softened
- 3 ounces marshmallow creme
- 1/2 cup reduced-fat vanilla yogurt
- 1 large apple , cut into chunks
- 1 cup sliced strawberries
- 1/2 cup jicama , cut into matchsticks
- 1/2 cup mandarin orange segments
- 1/2 cup blueberries
- 1/2 cup chopped walnuts , toasted
- 8 cones flat bottomed ice cream cones

Directions:

1. Beat cream cheese, marshmallow creme, and vanilla yogurt together in a bowl until smooth.
2. Mix apple, strawberries, jicama, mandarin orange segments, blueberries, and walnuts in a sizable bowl.
3. Pour cream cheese mixture over fruit and toss to mix. Cover and refrigerate until well chilled.
4. Scoop fruit and cream cheese mixture into ice cream cones to serve.

Vanilla Ice Cream I Recipe

Ingredients:

- 1 cup white sugar
- 1 cup milk
- 2 large eggs
- 2 cups heavy cream
- 1 1/2 teaspoons vanilla extract
- 1 tablespoon fresh lemon juice

Directions:

1. Combine the cream, milk, and sugar in a bowl. Stir before sugar is totally dissolved. Stir in the vanilla and almond extract.
2. Add the cherries. Pour the mixture into an ice cream maker and churn based on the manufacturer's

instructions. Transfer to a freezer-safe container and freeze for at least 2 hours before serving

Ice Cream In A Bag

Ingredients:
- 1 cup half-and-half
- 2 tablespoons granulated sugar
- 1/2 teaspoon pure vanilla extract
- 3 cups ice
- 1/3 cup kosher salt
- toppings of your choice

Directions:
1. In a little resealable plastic bag, combine half-and-half, sugar, and vanilla. Push out excess air and seal. Into a big resealable plastic bag, combine ice and salt.
2. Place small bag in the bigger bag and shake vigorously, 7 to ten minutes, until ice cream has hardened. Remove from bag and revel in with your preferred ice cream toppings.

Pumpkin Ice Cream Recipe

Ingredients:
- 1 (15-ounce) can pumpkins
- 1 cup white sugar
- 1 teaspoon salt
- 1 teaspoon ground ginger
- 1 teaspoon ground cinnamon
- 1/2 teaspoon ground nutmeg
- 1 cup chopped pecans
- 1/2 gallon vanilla ice cream , softened
- 36 wafers vanilla wafers

Directions:
1. In a large bowl, combine pumpkin, sugar, salt, ginger, cinnamon and nutmeg and mix until well blended. Stir in pecans. Fold in ice cream.
2. Line a 9x13 inch dish or sealable plastic container with 18 cookies. Spread half the ice cream mixture over the cookies. Repeat layers. Freeze until firm.

Reese's N'ice Cream

Ingredients:
- 8 large ripe bananas. sliced into coins
- 1/2 cup smooth peanut butter smooth peanut butter, plus 1/4 c melted peanut butter
- 1 teaspoon pure vanilla extract
- 1 cup chopped reese's, plus more for topping
- 1/4 cup melted chocolate

Directions:
1. Freeze bananas until frozen, about 2 hours. In a food processor, blend together bananas, 1/2 cup peanut butter, and vanilla.
2. Pour mixture into a loaf pan and fold in Reese's. Drizzle top with melted chocolate and melted peanut butter then scatter more Reese's at the top. Freeze until solid, about 3 hour

Ice Cream Bonbon Pops

Ingredients:
- crushed popcorn
- 1 pint vanilla ice cream, or your favorite flavor
- about eighteen 4-inch lollipop sticks
- crushed candy , such as sno-caps, whoppers, skittles and m&m's

Directions:
1. Place 2 parchment paper-lined large plates in the freezer for quarter-hour. Disseminate crushed popcorn on a baking sheet.
2. Using an ice cream scoop and working quickly, scoop out 9 ice cream balls and place along with the popcorn. Return the pint of ice cream to the freezer so it doesn't melt. Roll the balls in the popcorn to coat, pressing to greatly help it adhere. Insert sticks into the centers of the balls, then transfer the bonbons to 1 of the frozen plates and transfer to the freezer.
3. Repeat with the candy and remaining ice cream and plate. Freeze the bonbons until they are completely firm, about thirty minutes.

Irish Cream Ice Cream Recipe

Ingredients:
- 2 cups half-and-half
- 1/2 cup white sugar

- 1/2 cup brown sugar
- 2 cups heavy whipping cream
- 1 tablespoon vanilla extract
- 1/2 cup irish cream liqueur

Directions:

1. Beat together half-and-half, white sugar, and brown sugar in a sizable bowl with an electric mixer on medium speed before sugars have dissolved.
2. Stir heavy cream and vanilla extract in to the mixture until smooth.
3. Pour the mixture into an ice cream maker and freeze according to manufacturer's instructions.
4. About 2 minutes prior to the end of freezing time, pour Irish cream liqueur in to the ice cream maker; permit the machine to complete freezing the ice cream.
5. Transfer ice cream right into a freezer-proof container with a tight lid and place in freezer until ice cream is hardened, at least 4 hours.

Peach-buttermilk Ice Cream

Ingredients:

- 1 1/2 pounds peaches (about 6 small), plus sliced peaches for serving
- 1 cup farm-fresh buttermilk
- 1 teaspoon grated lemons zest plus 2 tablespoons fresh lemon juice
- 6 large eggs yolks
- 2 cups heavy cream
- 1 cup sugar
- 1/8 teaspoon kosher salt
- 1 vanilla bean , split lengthwise, seeds scraped

Directions:

1. Bring a medium saucepan of water to a boil. Fill a huge bowl with ice water. Using a sharp paring knife, mark an X on the bottom of every peach. Add the peaches to the saucepan and blanch before skins start to peel away, 1 to 2 2 minutes. Transfer the peaches to the ice bath and let cool completely. Get rid of the saucepan.
2. Peel and chop the peaches. Transfer to a food processor and puree until smooth. Scrape into a huge bowl and whisk in the buttermilk, lemon zest and lemon juice. Cover and refrigerate until cold.

3. In a heatproof medium bowl, whisk the egg yolks. In the medium saucepan, simmer the cream with the sugar, salt and the vanilla bean and seeds over moderate heat, whisking occasionally, before sugar has dissolved, about five minutes. While whisking constantly, slowly stream half of the hot cream mixture in to the egg yolks. Pour the mixture back to the saucepan and cook over moderately low heat, whisking constantly, before custard is thick enough to coat the trunk of a spoon, 8 to ten minutes. Strain the custard through an excellent sieve set over a heatproof bowl and let cool to room temperature. Whisk in the chilled buttermilk-peach mixture. Press a sheet of plastic wrap directly onto the top of custard and refrigerate until cold, at least 3 hours.
4. Employed in 2 batches, freeze the ice cream base in an ice cream machine based on the manufacturer's instructions. Pack the ice cream into plastic containers and freeze until firm, at least 4 hours or overnight. Serve the ice cream topped with sliced peaches.

Frozen Strawberry Yogurt Recipe

Ingredients:

- 1 pound fresh strawberries
- 3/4 cup white sugar
- 1 tablespoon vanilla extract
- 1/4 cup half-and-half
- 1 (32-ounce) container plain yogurt

Directions:

1. Place strawberries, sugar, vanilla extract, and half-and-half in a blender; puree until smooth. Add yogurt and pulse until combined.
2. Pour the mixture into an ice cream maker and freeze according to manufacturer's instructions. Transfer frozen yogurt to a lidded plastic container. Cover surface with plastic wrap and seal. For best results, let it ripen in the freezer for at least 2 hours or overnight before serving.

Hazelnut Gelato Recipe

Ingredients:

- 2 cups whole milk
- 1 cup heavy whipping cream

- 1/3 cup white sugar
- 4 large eggs yolks egg yolks
- 1/3 cup white sugar
- 1/2 cup chocolate hazelnut spread
- 2 tablespoons instant espresso powder
- 1/2 teaspoon vanilla extract

Directions:

1. Combine milk, cream, and 1/3 cup sugar in a saucepan over medium heat; cook and stir until sugar dissolves, 3 to 5 minutes.

2. Beat egg yolks and 1/3 cup sugar together in a bowl until mixture is light yellow, about 4 minutes. Stir 1/2 cup milk mixture into egg mixture until smooth; pour into the remaining milk mixture in the saucepan, stirring continuously.

3. Cook, stirring continuously, until mixture thickens enough to coat the back of a metal spoon, 8 to 10 minutes; remove from heat.

4. Stir chocolate hazelnut spread, espresso powder, and vanilla extract into milk mixture until well combined; pour through a mesh strainer into a bowl. Refrigerate mixture until cold, about 3 hours.

5. Pour milk mixture into an ice cream maker and freeze according to manufacturer's instructions.

Fig Ice Cream Recipe

Ingredients:

- 2 cups dried figs
- 2 tablespoons white sugar
- 1 teaspoon lemon juice
- 2 1/2 cups half-and-half
- 1/2 cup white sugar
- 3 large eggs yolks egg yolks
- 1 teaspoon salt
- 1 cup reduced-fat sour cream
- 1 teaspoon vanilla extract

Directions:

1. Soak figs in a plate of water until softened, three to four 4 hours. Drain figs and chop.

2. Combine chopped figs, 2 tablespoons sugar, and lemon juice in a saucepan over medium heat; cook and stir until sugar is dissolved and figs begin to break down, 4 to 5 minutes. Remove saucepan from heat and cool to room temperature, 15 to 20 minutes. Cover saucepan with a lid and refrigerate.

3. Heat half-and-half in a heavy saucepan over medium-high heat until hot however, not boiling, 5 to 6 minutes. Remove saucepan from heat.

4. Whisk 1/2 cup sugar, egg yolks, and salt together in a bowl until smooth. Temper egg mixture by drizzling 1 to 2 2 tablespoons half-and-half into egg mixture, while consistently whisking egg mixture until slightly warmed. Pour egg mixture into half-and-half and return saucepan to medium-low heat; cook, whisking constantly, until custard is smooth and thickened, about five minutes.

5. Place saucepan with custard in the refrigerator, stirring occasionally, until chilled, about thirty minutes. Stir sour cream and vanilla extract into chilled custard. Cover saucepan and chill custard completely, at least 3 hours.

6. Process custard within an ice cream maker according to manufacturer's instructions. Stir fig mixture into ice cream within the last 5 minutes of processing. Transfer fig ice cream to a container and freeze until solid.

Cherry Ice Cream Recipe

Ingredients:

- 1/4 cup cherry juice concentrate
- 1/2 cup fat free milk
- 1 cup vanilla low-fat yogurt
- 1 cup heavy cream
- 1/2 cup white sugar
- 1 pinch salt
- 1 cup frozen dark sweet cherries
- 2 teaspoons almond extract

Directions:

1. Place the cherry juice, milk, yogurt, and heavy cream into the plate of a blender. Add the sugar, salt, cherries, and almond extract. Puree until only small bits of the cherries remain.

2. Pour right into a 1 1/2 quart ice cream maker and freeze according to manufacturer's directions.

Strawberry Rosewater Ice Cream Recipe

Ingredients:

- 1 1/2 cups fresh strawberries , hulled
- 1/3 cup white sugar

- 3 eaches eggs yolks, beaten
- 1/2 pint milk
- 1/4 teaspoon salt
- 1/3 cup white sugar
- 1 pint heavy cream
- 1/4 cup rosewater

Directions:

1. Combine the strawberries and 1/3 cup sugar in a bowl; mash as well as a potato masher. Store the mixture in the refrigerator while preparing all of those other recipe.

2. Stir together the egg yolks, milk, salt and 1/3 cup sugar in a saucepan over medium heat. Heat to 175 degrees F (80 degrees C), making sure the mixture will not boil; transfer to a chilled bowl and move to the refrigerator to cool, stirring occasionally. Once cooled, stir in the cream, rosewater, and strawberry mixture.

3. Fill an ice cream maker with the mixture, and freeze based on the manufacturer's instructions.

Cherry Cheesecake Ice Cream

Ingredients:

- 3 cups cold heavy cream
- 1 14 cans -oz. sweetened condensed milk
- 1 teaspoon pure vanilla extract
- 1 cup hand crushed graham crackers (about 4 whole crackers), plus more for garnish
- 1 cup cherry pie filling

Directions:

1. In a sizable bowl utilizing a hand mixer, beat cream until stiff peaks form, 2-3 three minutes. Fold in sweetened condensed milk and vanilla until fully incorporated, then fold in crushed graham crackers.

2. Transfer half the mixture to a 9"-x-5" loaf pan. Dollop 1/2 cup pie filling over top, then swirl with a knife.

3. Add remaining cream mixture, then swirl in remaining 1/2 cup pie filling. Top with graham crackers. Freeze until firm, at least 8 hours, covering lightly with plastic wrap after 4 hours. Let soften ten minutes before scooping and serving.

Chocolate Frosty Recipe

Ingredients:

- 1 quart chocolate milk
- 1 (14-ounce) can sweetened condensed milk
- 1 (8-ounce) container frozen whipped topping (such as cool whip®), thawed

Directions:

1. Mix chocolate milk, sweetened condensed milk, and whipped topping in a large bowl.

2. Pour mixture into an ice cream maker and freeze according to manufacturer's instructions.

Peanut Butter-banana V'ice Cream

Ingredients:

- 4 very ripe bananas
- 1/4 cup peanut butter (smooth or chunky)
- 1 tablespoon coconut oils
- 1/2 teaspoon ground cinnamon
- 1/4 teaspoon grated nutmeg
- pinch of kosher salt

Directions:

1. Slice bananas into 1/4"-thick rounds and devote a ziptop plastic bag. Lay the slices flat in a single layer in the freezer therefore the rounds freeze individually rather than in a large clump.

2. Freeze the bananas for at least 2 hours and up to overnight. Place the frozen bananas, peanut butter, coconut oil, cinnamon, nutmeg, and salt in a food processor or blender and let sit for 2 or 3 three minutes. Then puree until creamy and smooth. If you like a frozen yogurt consistency, then serve it up.

3. If you like a firmer ice cream experience, spoon it right into a container and freeze for approximately an hour.

Chai Tea Ice Cream Recipe

Ingredients:

- 3 cups whole milk , or more to taste
- 3 cups heavy whipping cream
- 3 cups white sugar
- 4 cinnamon sticks cinnamon sticks
- 4 tablespoons indian-style plain black tea
- 3 tablespoons garam masala (indian spice blend)

- 10 eaches black peppercorns
- 6 eaches cardamom pods
- 2 eaches whole star anise pods
- 1 teaspoon ground nutmeg
- 1 tablespoon vanilla extract
- 1 cup chopped semisweet chocolate

Directions:

1. Mix dairy, whipping cream, sugar, cinnamon sticks, tea, garam masala, peppercorns, cardamom pods, anise pods, and nutmeg together in a saucepan; bring to a simmer and cook for 20 minutes.

2. Strain mixture through a colander into a sizable bowl. Soon add up to 1 cup more milk to cut spice level and sweetness to your liking.

3. Pour milk mixture into an ice cream maker and churn according to the manufacturer's instructions.

4. Stir chocolate into the churned milk mixture and freeze, stirring occasionally, until soft and creamy, 4 to 5 hours.

FRUITILICIOUS ICE CREAM

Blueberry Chocolate Vegan Soft Serve Ice Cream

Servings: 9
Cooking Time: 10 Minutes
Ingredients:
- 3/4 cup water
- 1 1/4 cups full fat coconut milk or coconut cream (as thick as possible)
- 2/3 cup organic cane sugar
- 2/3 cup unsweetened cocoa powder
- 1/4 tsp sea salt
- 6 ounces vegan dark chocolate, finely chopped
- 1/2 tsp pure vanilla extract
- 1/2 cup blueberries

Directions:
1. NOTE: Freeze your ice cream bowl for at least 24hrs prior to starting!
2. Put the first 5 ingredients in a large saucepan, and heat it on medium-high heat. Mix the ingredients together using a whisk. Allow the mixture to come to a low boil. Continue to whisk often, and remain cooking on a low boil for 1 minute.
3. Take the pan off the heat, and mix in the chocolate and vanilla extract using the whisk. Continue to mix until the chocolate is melted.
4. Place the mixture in a blender with the blueberries, and blend on high speed for about 30 seconds or until the blueberries are pureed.
5. Allow the mixture to cool
6. Pour the ingredients into your ice cream maker, and let it churn for 25 minutes.
7. Serve immediately.

Astounding Apricot Almond Ice Cream

Servings: 6
Cooking Time: 2 Hours 50 Minutes
Ingredients:
- 2 cups heavy cream
- 1 cup milk
- 3/4 cup sugar
- 1 teaspoon vanilla extract
- 1 cup sliced apricots
- ½ cup chopped almonds

Directions:
1. Refer to note at the beginning of the chapter about freezing bowl.
2. Puree the apricots in a food processor or blender.
3. Place the milk and cream in a bowl, and mix them together until well combined. Use a whisk to mix in the sugar. Continue to whisk for about 4 minutes until the sugar dissolves. Then mix in the vanilla extract, and apricot puree.
4. Pour the ingredients into your ice cream maker, and let it churn for 25 minutes. About 5 minutes before the ice cream is finished churning, add in the almonds.
5. Put the ice cream in an airtight container and place in the freezer for around 2 hours. Allow the ice cream to thaw for 15 minutes before serving.

Apricot Honey Gelato

Servings: 4-6
Cooking Time: 2 Hours 35 Minutes
Ingredients:
- 1/2 cup heavy cream
- 2 cups milk
- 3/4 cup sugar
- 1 tablespoon vanilla extract
- 1 cup sliced apricot
- 1/4 cup honey

Directions:
1. Refer to note at the beginning of the chapter about freezing bowl.
2. Puree the apricots in a food processor or blender.
3. Place the milk and cream in a bowl, and mix them together until well combined. Use a whisk to mix in the sugar. Continue to whisk for about 4 minutes until the sugar dissolves. Then mix in the vanilla extract honey and apricot puree.
4. Pour the ingredients into your ice cream maker, and let it churn for 25 minutes.
5. Put the gelato in an airtight container and place in the freezer for up to 2 hours, until desired consistency is reached.

Juicy Strawberry Honey Frozen Yogurt

Servings: 1 Quart
Cooking Time: 2 Hours 35 Minutes
Ingredients:

- 1 quart container full-fat plain yogurt
- ¼ teaspoon salt
- 1 cup sugar
- 1 teaspoon vanilla extract
- 8 ounces strawberries
- 1/4 cup honey

Directions:
1. Refer to note at the beginning of the chapter about freezing bowl.
2. Puree the strawberries in a food processor or blender.
3. Place the yogurt in a bowl. Use a whisk to mix in the sugar and salt. Continue to whisk for about 4 minutes until the sugar dissolves. Then mix in the vanilla extract, honey and strawberry puree.
4. Pour the ingredients into your ice cream maker, and let it churn for 25 minutes.
5. Put the frozen yogurt in an airtight container and place in the freezer for at least 2 hours, until desired consistency is reached.

Double Cherry Chocolate Milkshake

Servings: 6
Cooking Time: 25 Minutes
Ingredients:

- 2 cups heavy cream
- 1 cup milk
- 3/4 cup sugar
- 1 teaspoon vanilla extract
- 1 cup cherry juice
- ¼ cup semi-sweet chocolate chips

Directions:
1. Refer to note at the beginning of the chapter about freezing bowl.
2. Place the milk and cream in a bowl, and mix them together until well combined. Use a whisk to mix in the sugar. Continue to whisk for about 4 minutes until the sugar dissolves. Then mix in the vanilla extract, and cherry juice.
3. Pour the ingredients into your ice cream maker, and let it churn for 10-15 minutes, until desired

consistency is reached. About 5 minutes before the ice cream is finished churning, add in the chocolate chips.
4. Serve immediately.

Chocolate Raspberry Pistachio Vegan Gelato

Servings: 4
Cooking Time: 2 Hours 35 Minutes
Ingredients:

- 2 cups shelled, roasted, salted pistachios
- 1 can coconut milk
- 1/2 cup arrowroot
- ¾ cup sugar
- 1 teaspoon lime juice
- 4 ounces chopped vegan chocolate
- 1/4 cup raspberries

Directions:
1. NOTE: Freeze your ice cream bowl for at least 24hrs prior to starting!
2. Pulse the pistachios in a food processor for about 3 minutes
3. Place all ingredients EXCEPT the chocolate in a blender. Blend on high speed until smooth.
4. Pour the mixture into your ice cream maker, and let it churn for 25 minutes. About 5 minutes before the ice cream is done churning add the chocolate to your ice cream maker.
5. Put the gelato in an airtight container and place in the freezer for up to 2 hours, until desired consistency is reached.

Grapelicious Ice Cream

Servings: 6
Cooking Time: 2 Hours 50 Minutes
Ingredients:

- 2 cups heavy cream
- 1 cup milk
- 3/4 cup sugar
- 1 teaspoon vanilla extract
- 2 cans (12 ounces) frozen grape juice concentrate
- juice of 3 lemons

Directions:

1. Refer to note at the beginning of the chapter about freezing bowl.
2. Place the milk and cream in a bowl, and mix them together until well combined. Use a whisk to mix in the sugar. Continue to whisk for about 4 minutes until the sugar dissolves. Then mix in the vanilla extract, grape juice, and lemon juice.
3. Pour the ingredients into your ice cream maker, and let it churn for 25 minutes.
4. Put the ice cream in an airtight container and place in the freezer for around 2 hours. Allow the ice cream to thaw for 15 minutes before serving.

Blackberry Lemon Coconut Vegan Frozen Yogurt

Servings: 1 Quart
Cooking Time: 2 Hours 35 Minutes
Ingredients:
- 2 cups coconut yogurt
- 1/4 cup sugar or maple syrup
- 1/2 teaspoon vanilla extract
- 1/4 cup shredded coconut
- ½ cup blackberries
- 1 lemon

Directions:
1. NOTE: Freeze your ice cream bowl for at least 24hrs prior to starting!
2. Puree the blackberries and lemon in a food processor or blender.
3. Place the yogurt in a bowl. Use a whisk to mix in the sugar. Continue to whisk for about 4 minutes until the sugar dissolves. Then mix in the vanilla extract, and blackberry puree.
4. Pour the ingredients into your ice cream maker, and let it churn for 25 minutes. About 5 minutes before the ice cream is done churning add the shredded coconut to your ice cream maker.
5. Put the frozen yogurt in an airtight container and place in the freezer for at least 2 hours, until desired consistency is reached.

Lemon Lime Milkshake

Servings: 6
Cooking Time: 25 Minutes

Ingredients:
- 2 cups heavy cream
- 1 cup milk
- 3/4 cup sugar
- 1 teaspoon vanilla extract
- ¼ cup lime juice
- ¼ cup lemon juice
- Zest of one lemon
- Zest of one lime

Directions:
1. Refer to note at the beginning of the chapter about freezing bowl.
2. Place the milk and cream in a bowl, and mix them together until well combined. Use a whisk to mix in the sugar. Continue to whisk for about 4 minutes until the sugar dissolves. Then mix in the vanilla extract, juice, and zest.
3. Pour the ingredients into your ice cream maker, and let it churn for 10-15 minutes, until desired consistency is reached.
4. Serve immediately.

Kickin' Kiwi Lime Ice Cream

Servings: 6
Cooking Time: 2 Hours 50 Minutes
Ingredients:
- 2 cups heavy cream
- 1 cup milk
- 3/4 cup sugar
- 1/2 teaspoon vanilla extract
- ½ teaspoon salt
- 1 kiwi, peeled
- Juice of one and a half limes

Directions:
1. Refer to note at the beginning of the chapter about freezing bowl.
2. Puree the kiwi in a food processor or blender.
3. Place the milk and cream in a bowl, and mix them together until well combined. Use a whisk to mix in the sugar and salt. Continue to whisk for about 4 minutes until the sugar and salt dissolves. Then mix in the vanilla extract, lime juice, and kiwi puree.
4. Pour the ingredients into your ice cream maker, and let it churn for 25 minutes.

5. Put the ice cream in an airtight container and place in the freezer for around 2 hours. Allow the ice cream to thaw for 15 minutes before serving.

Peanut Butter White Chocolate Soft Serve Ice Cream

Servings: 6
Cooking Time: 40 Minutes
Ingredients:
- 2 cups heavy cream
- 1 cup milk
- 3/4 cup sugar
- 1 Tbs. vanilla extract
- 1/2 cup peanut butter slightly melted
- 2 ounces semi-sweet chocolate

Directions:
1. NOTE: Freeze your ice cream bowl for at least 24hrs prior to starting!
2. Melt the chocolate in a medium sauce pan on low heat. Allow the chocolate to cool a bit.
3. While the chocolate is cooling, place the milk and cream in a bowl, and mix them together until well combined. Use a whisk to mix in the sugar. Continue to whisk for about 4 minutes until the sugar dissolves. Mix in the vanilla extract. Then whisk in the peanut butter, and then the chocolate.
4. Pour the ingredients into your ice cream maker, and let it churn for 25 minutes.
5. Serve immediately.

Vanilla Apple Cinnamon Ice Cream

Servings: 6
Cooking Time: 2 Hours 50 Minutes
Ingredients:
- 2 cups heavy cream
- 1 cup milk
- 3/4 cup sugar
- 1 teaspoon vanilla extract
- 1 teaspoon ground cinnamon
- 2 large apples peeled, cored, and sliced
- 1/4 cup chopped walnuts

Directions:
1. Refer to note at the beginning of the chapter about freezing bowl.

2. Puree the apples in a food processor or blender.
3. Place the milk and cream in a bowl, and mix them together until well combined. Use a whisk to mix in the sugar. Continue to whisk for about 4 minutes until the sugar dissolves. Then mix in the vanilla extract, cinnamon, and apple puree.
4. Pour the ingredients into your ice cream maker, and let it churn for 25 minutes. About 5 minutes before the ice cream is finished churning, add in the walnuts and several drops of vanilla!.
5. Put the ice cream in an airtight container and place in the freezer for around 2 hours. Allow the ice cream to thaw for 15 minutes before serving.

Orange Chocolate Almond Vegan Ice Cream

Servings: 9
Cooking Time: 10 Minutes
Ingredients:
- 3/4 cup water
- 1 1/4 cups full fat coconut milk or coconut cream (as thick as possible)
- 2/3 cup organic cane sugar
- 2/3 cup unsweetened cocoa powder
- 1/4 tsp sea salt
- 6 ounces vegan dark chocolate, finely chopped
- 1/2 tsp pure vanilla extract
- ½ cup chopped almonds
- ½ tsp orange extract

Directions:
1. NOTE: Freeze your ice cream bowl for at least 24hrs prior to starting!
2. Put the first 5 ingredients in a large saucepan, and heat it on medium-high heat. Mix the ingredients together using a whisk. Allow the mixture to come to a low boil. Continue to whisk often, and remain cooking on a low boil for 1 minute.
3. Take the pan off the heat, and mix in the chocolate and vanilla extract using the whisk. Continue to mix until the chocolate is melted.
4. Place the mixture in a blender, blend on high (30 seconds) and allow the mixture to cool.
5. Pour the ingredients into your ice cream maker, and let it churn for 25 minutes. About 5 minutes before the ice cream is done churning.

6. Put the ice cream in an airtight container and place in the freezer for around 2 hours. Allow the ice cream to thaw for 15 minutes before serving.

Big Blueberry Chocolate Gelato

Servings: 4-6
Cooking Time: 2 Hours 35 Minutes
Ingredients:
- 1/2 cup heavy cream
- 2 cups milk
- 3/4 cup sugar
- 1 teaspoon vanilla extract
- 1 cup blueberries
- ½ cup finely chopped semi-sweet

Directions:
1. Refer to note at the beginning of the chapter about freezing bowl.
2. Puree the bananas in a food processor or blender.
3. Place the milk and cream in a bowl, and mix them together until well combined. Use a whisk to mix in the sugar. Continue to whisk for about 4 minutes until the sugar dissolves. Then mix in the vanilla extract and banana puree.
4. Pour the ingredients into your ice cream maker, and let it churn for 25 minutes. About 5 minutes before the ice cream is done churning add the chocolate to your ice cream maker.
5. Put the gelato in an airtight container and place in the freezer for up to 2 hours, until desired consistency is reached.

Peaches And Cream Soft Serve Ice Cream

Servings: 6
Cooking Time: 35 Minutes
Ingredients:
- 2 cups heavy cream
- 1 cup milk
- 3/4 cup sugar
- 1 Tbs. vanilla extract
- 1 cup sliced peaches

Directions:
1. Refer to note at the beginning of the chapter about freezing bowl.

2. Puree the peaches in a food processor or blender.
3. Place the milk and cream in a bowl, and mix them together until well combined. Use a whisk to mix in the sugar. Continue to whisk for about 4 minutes until the sugar dissolves. Then mix in the vanilla extract. Then mix in the peaches.
4. Pour the ingredients into your ice cream maker, and let it churn for 25 minutes.
5. Serve immediately.

Kickin' Key Lime Sorbet

Servings: 4
Cooking Time: 3 Hours
Ingredients:
- 3 cups cold water
- 2 ¼ cup fresh key lime juice
- 2 3/4 cup sugar
- 1 tablespoon lime zest

Directions:
1. Refer to note at the beginning of the chapter about freezing bowl.
2. Mix together the water and sugar in a large sauce pan on medium heat. Allow the mixture to come to a boil. Then lower to low heat, and let the mixture simmer until the sugar dissolve. Allow the mixture to cool completely.
3. Mix the lime juice and zest with the cooled mixture.
4. Pour the ingredients into your ice cream maker, and let it churn for 25-30 minutes.
5. Place in an airtight container for up to 2 hours, until desired consistency is reached.

Chocolate Cherry Cocoa Banana Vegan Milkshake

Servings: 9
Cooking Time: 10 Minutes
Ingredients:
- 3/4 cup water
- 1 1/4 cups full fat coconut milk or coconut cream (as thick as possible)
- 2/3 cup organic cane sugar
- 2/3 cup unsweetened cocoa powder

- 1/4 tsp sea salt
- 6 oz. vegan dark chocolate, finely chopped
- 1/2 tsp pure vanilla extract
- ¼ cup sliced frozen bananas
- ¼ cup cherries (cut up fine)
- 1 tbsp. cinnamon

Directions:

1. NOTE: Freeze your ice cream bowl for at least 24hrs prior to starting!
2. Put the first 5 ingredients in a large saucepan, and heat it on medium-high heat. Mix the ingredients together using a whisk. Allow the mixture to come to a low boil. Continue to whisk often, and remain cooking on a low boil for 1 minute.
3. Take the pan off the heat, and mix in the chocolate and vanilla extract using the whisk. Continue to mix until the chocolate is melted. Add cherries and cinnamon.
4. Place the mixture in a blender with the bananas, and blend on high speed for about 30 seconds, then allow the mixture to cool
5. Pour the ingredients into your ice cream maker, and let it churn for 10-15 minutes, until desired consistency is reached and serve immediately.

"bursting" Blueberry Maple Syrup Soft Serve Ice Cream

Servings: 6
Cooking Time: 35 Minutes
Ingredients:

- 2 cups heavy cream
- 1 cup milk
- 3/4 cup sugar
- 1 Tbs. vanilla extract
- 1 cup blueberries
- ¼ cup maple syrup

Directions:

1. Refer to note at the beginning of the chapter about freezing bowl.
2. Puree the blueberries in a food processor or blender.
3. Place the milk and cream in a bowl, and mix them together until well combined. Use a whisk to mix in the sugar. Continue to whisk for about 4 minutes until the sugar dissolves. Then mix in the

vanilla extract. Then mix in the blueberries, and maple syrup.
4. Pour the ingredients into your ice cream maker, and let it churn for 25 minutes.
5. Serve immediately.

Tropical Mango Soft Serve Ice Cream

Servings: 6
Cooking Time: 35 Minutes
Ingredients:

- 2 cups heavy cream
- 1 cup milk
- 3/4 cup sugar
- 1 Tbs. vanilla extract
- 1 cup pureed mango (about 2.5 mangos)
- Juice of 1 lime

Directions:

1. Refer to note at the beginning of the chapter about freezing bowl.
2. Puree the mangos with the lime juice in a food processor or blender.
3. Place the milk and cream in a bowl, and mix them together until well combined. Use a whisk to mix in the sugar. Continue to whisk for about 4 minutes until the sugar dissolves. Then mix in the vanilla extract. Then mix in the mango puree.
4. Pour the ingredients into your ice cream maker, and let it churn for 25 minutes.
5. Serve immediately.

Bursting Banana Nut Gelato

Servings: 4-6
Cooking Time: 2 Hours 35 Minutes
Ingredients:

- 1/2 cup heavy cream
- 2 cups milk
- 3/4 cup sugar
- 1 tablespoon vanilla extract
- 1 cup sliced banana
- ½ cup chopped walnuts

Directions:

1. Refer to note at the beginning of the chapter about freezing bowl.

2. Puree the bananas in a food processor or blender.

3. Place the milk and cream in a bowl, and mix them together until well combined. Use a whisk to mix in the sugar. Continue to whisk for about 4 minutes until the sugar dissolves. Then mix in the vanilla extract and banana puree.

4. Pour the ingredients into your ice cream maker, and let it churn for 25 minutes. About 5 minutes before the ice cream is done churning add the walnuts to your ice cream maker.

5. Put the gelato in an airtight container and place in the freezer for up to 2 hours, until desired consistency is reached.

Pineapple Strawberries N Cream Tofu Vegan Ice Cream

Servings: Makes 1 Quart
Cooking Time: 35 Minutes
Ingredients:
- 1 pound silken tofu
- ½ cup plus 2 tablespoons organic or granulated sugar
- ½ teaspoon kosher salt
- 1 vanilla bean, split lengthwise
- ¾ cup refined coconut oil, melted, cooled slightly
- ½ cup sliced strawberries
- ½ cup pineapple

Directions:
1. NOTE: Freeze your ice cream bowl for at least 24hrs prior to starting!

2. Put the first 3 ingredients in a blender. Then add in the vanilla bean seeds, pineapples and strawberries. Puree the mixture until its smooth, around 15 seconds. Turn the blender to medium speed, and slowly drizzle in the coconut oil. Blend the mixture until its thick, but don't over blend it.

3. Pour the ingredients into your ice cream maker, and let it churn for 25 minutes.

4. Put the ice cream in an airtight container and place in the freezer for around 2 hours. Allow the ice cream to thaw for 15 minutes before serving.

Raspberry Pumpkin Spice Vegan Soy Frozen Yogurt

Servings: 1 Quart
Cooking Time: 2 Hours 30 Minutes
Ingredients:
- 2 ¾ cups unsweetened plain soy yogurt
- 1¼ raspberry jam
- 1 tbsp. pumpkin spice

Directions:
1. NOTE: Freeze your ice cream bowl for at least 24hrs prior to starting!

2. Place the yogurt in a bowl and mix in the jam. Use a hand mixer to beat the mixture for 5 minutes.

3. Pour the ingredients into your ice cream maker, and let it churn for 25 minutes.

4. Put the frozen yogurt in an airtight container and place in the freezer for at least 2 hours, until desired consistency is reached.

Chocolate Peppermint Banana Vegan Milkshake

Servings: 9
Cooking Time: 10 Minutes
Ingredients:
- 3/4 cup water
- 1 1/4 cups full fat coconut milk or coconut cream (as thick as possible)
- 2/3 cup organic cane sugar
- 2/3 cup unsweetened cocoa powder
- 1/4 tsp sea salt
- 6 ounces vegan dark chocolate, finely chopped
- 11/2 tsp peppermint extract
- ½ cup sliced frozen bananas

Directions:
1. NOTE: Freeze your ice cream bowl for at least 24hrs prior to starting!

2. Put the first 5 ingredients in a large saucepan, and heat it on medium-high heat. Mix the ingredients together using a whisk. Allow the mixture to come to a low boil. Continue to whisk often, and remain cooking on a low boil for 1 minute.

3. Take the pan off the heat, and mix in the chocolate and mint extract using the whisk. Continue to mix until the chocolate is melted.

4. Place mixture in a blender with the bananas, and blend on high speed for about 30 seconds.

5. Allow the mixture to cool

6. Pour the ingredients into your ice cream maker, and let it churn for 10-15 minutes, until desired consistency is reached.

7. Serve immediately.

Nutella & Bananas Soft Serve Ice Cream

Servings: 6
Cooking Time: 35 Minutes
Ingredients:
- 1 cup sliced Bananas
- 6 tbs. Nutella
- 2 cups heavy cream
- 1 cup milk
- 3/4 cup sugar
- 1 Tbs. vanilla extract

Directions:
1. NOTE: Freeze your ice cream bowl for at least 24hrs prior to starting!

2. Place the milk and cream in a bowl, and mix them together until well combined. Use a whisk to mix in the sugar. Continue to whisk for about 4 minutes until the sugar dissolves. Then mix in the vanilla extract.

3. Place all the ingredients in a food processor or blender, and puree.

4. Pour the ingredients into your ice cream maker, and let it churn for 25 minutes.

5. Serve immediately.

Caribbean Pineapple Sorbet

Servings: 9
Cooking Time: 2 Hours 40 Minutes
Ingredients:
- 1 diced, peeled, and cored small pineapple
- 2 tablespoons lemon juice
- 1 cup plus 2 tablespoons sugar

Directions:
1. Refer to note at the beginning of the chapter about freezing bowl.

2. Puree the pineapple and lemon juice in a food processor or blender. Then add in the sugar and puree until the sugar dissolves.

3. Pour the ingredients into your ice cream maker, and let it churn for 25-30 minutes.

4. Place in an airtight container for up to 2 hours, until desired consistency is reached.

Basil Chocolate Vegan Soft Serve Ice Cream

Servings: 9
Cooking Time: 10 Minutes
Ingredients:
- 3/4 cup water
- 1 1/4 cups full fat coconut milk or coconut cream (as thick as possible)
- 2/3 cup organic cane sugar
- 2/3 cup unsweetened cocoa powder
- 1/4 tsp sea salt
- 6 ounces vegan dark chocolate, finely chopped
- 1/2 tsp pure vanilla extract
- ¼ cup basil (pulverized)

Directions:
1. NOTE: Freeze your ice cream bowl for at least 24hrs prior to starting!

2. Put the first 5 ingredients in a large saucepan, and heat it on medium-high heat. Mix the ingredients together using a whisk. Allow the mixture to come to a low boil. Continue to whisk often, and remain cooking on a low boil for 1 minute.

3. Take the pan off the heat, and mix in the chocolate and vanilla extract using the whisk. Continue to mix until the chocolate is melted then add the basil.

4. Place the mixture in a blender, and blend on high speed for about 30 seconds.

5. Allow the mixture to cool

6. Pour the ingredients into your ice cream maker, and let it churn for 25 minutes.

7. Serve immediately.

Lemon Chocolate Blueberry Vegan Gelato

Servings: Makes 3 Cups
Cooking Time: 2 Hours 35 Minutes

Ingredients:
- 1 ½ cup refrigerated coconut cream
- 1 cup cut up lemons
- 3 tablespoons cocoa powder
- 1/2 teaspoon salt
- ½ cup blueberries

Directions:
1. NOTE: Freeze your ice cream bowl for at least 24hrs prior to starting!
2. Place all ingredients EXCEPT the blueberries in a blender. Blend on high speed until smooth.
3. Pour the mixture into your ice cream maker, and let it churn for 25 minutes. About 5 minutes before the ice cream is done churning add the blueberries to your ice cream maker.
4. Put the gelato in an airtight container and place in the freezer for up to 2 hours, until desired consistency is reached.

Pulsating Pomegranate Mint Frozen Yogurt

Servings: 1 Quart

Cooking Time: 2 Hours 35 Minutes

Ingredients:
- 1 quart container full-fat plain yogurt
- ¼ teaspoon salt
- 1 cup sugar
- 1 tablespoon mint extract
- 1 cup 100% pomegranate juice
- 1/2 cup semi-sweet chocolate chips

Directions:
1. Refer to note at the beginning of the chapter about freezing bowl.
2. Place the yogurt in a bowl. Use a whisk to mix in the sugar and salt. Continue to whisk for about 4 minutes until the sugar dissolves. Then mix in the mint extract, and pomegranate juice.
3. Pour the ingredients into your ice cream maker, and let it churn for 25 minutes. About 5 minutes before the ice cream is done churning add the chocolate chips to your ice cream maker.
4. Put the frozen yogurt in an airtight container and place in the freezer for at least 2 hours, until desired consistency is reached.

SIMPLE ICE CREAM

S'mores Camp Fire Frozen Yogurt

Servings: 1 Quart

Cooking Time: 2 Hours 35 Minutes

Ingredients:

- 1 quart container full-fat plain yogurt
- ¼ teaspoon salt
- 1 cup sugar
- 1 teaspoon vanilla extract
- 3 large graham crackers
- 4 ounces chopped semi-sweet chocolate
- ½ cup mini marshmallows
- 1 tsp smoke flavor extract

Directions:

1. NOTE: Freeze your ice cream bowl for at least 24hrs prior to starting!

2. Place the yogurt in a bowl. Use a whisk to mix in the sugar and salt. Continue to whisk for about 4 minutes until the sugar dissolves. Then mix in the vanilla and smoke flavored extract.

3. Place the graham crackers in a food processor, and process until the crackers are no bigger than chocolate chips. If you don't have a food processor place the crackers in a large resealable plastic bag, and seal it shut. Use your hands, a mallet, or a rolling pin to crush the cookies.

4. Pour the ingredients into your ice cream maker, and let it churn for 25 minutes. About 5 minutes before the ice cream is done churning add the chocolate, graham crackers, and marshmallows to your ice cream maker.

5. Put the frozen yogurt in an airtight container and place in the freezer for at least 2 hours, until desired consistency is reached.

Mango Ice Cream

Servings: 10

Cooking Time: 15 Minutes

Ingredients:

- 3 cups whole milk
- 1 cup sugar
- 8 egg yolks
- A pinch of salt
- ¼ cup mango puree
- 3 tablespoons dried mango, chopped

Directions:

1. Add the milk and sugar in a saucepan and heat over medium low flame. Simmer for 3 minutes or until the sugar dissolves. Remove from the heat.

2. In a bowl, whisk in the egg yolks. Drizzle ½ cup of the warm milk into the egg yolks while whisking constantly to form a smooth mixture. Whisk the egg mixture back into the pot. Add the salt.

3. Turn on the heat to medium low and cook until the mixture starts to thicken. Constantly stir while cooking. Add the mango puree last.

4. Turn off the heat and strain the mixture to remove lumps. Allow the milk to cool at room temperature. Place in the fridge to chill for 2 hours.

5. Turn on the Hamilton Beach and pour the mixture in. Churn for 15 minutes.

6. Five minutes before the time ends, add the dried mango.

7. Transfer to an airtight container.

8. Place in the fridge to completely cool.

Nutrition Info: Calories per serving:154 ; Protein: 4.3g; Carbs: 21.2g; Fat: 5.8g Sugar: 20.4g

Island Coconut Banana Sorbet

Servings: 4-8

Cooking Time: 2 Hours 40 Minutes

Ingredients:

- 3 peeled, mashed bananas
- 2-4 tablespoons honey to taste
- 1 1/2 cups light coconut milk
- 1 teaspoon vanilla extract

Directions:

1. Refer to note at the beginning of the chapter about freezing bowl.

2. Puree all ingredients in a food processor or blender. Taste, and add more honey if desired.

3. Pour the ingredients into your ice cream maker, and let it churn for 25-30 minutes.

4. Place in an airtight container for up to 2 hours, until desired consistency is reached.

Malted Milk Chocolate Ice Cream

Servings: 8
Cooking Time: 25 Minutes
Ingredients:
- 1 ¾ cups heavy cream
- 1 cup whole milk
- 2/3 cup malted milk powder
- ½ cup sugar
- A pinch of salt
- 6 egg yolks
- 6 ounces milk chocolate, chopped
- ½ cup mini Cadbury eggs, chopped

Directions:
1. Add the cream, milk, sugar, and salt in a saucepan and heat over medium low flame. Simmer for 3 minutes. Remove from the stove.
2. In a bowl, whisk in the egg yolks. Drizzle ½ cup of the warm milk into the egg yolks while whisking constantly to form a smooth mixture. Whisk the egg mixture back into the pot.
3. Turn on the heat to medium low and cook until the mixture starts to thicken. Constantly stir while cooking.
4. Turn off the heat and strain the mixture to remove lumps. Allow to cool at room temperature. Place in the fridge to chill for 2 hours.
5. Turn on the Hamilton Beach and pour the mixture in. Churn for 15 minutes.
6. Before the churning time ends, add the chopped milk chocolate and Cadbury eggs.
7. Transfer to an airtight container.
8. Place in the fridge to completely cool.
Nutrition Info: Calories per serving: 210; Protein: 5g; Carbs: 22g; Fat: 12g Sugar: 17g

Cinnamon Chocolate Chip Soft Serve Ice Cream

Servings: 6
Cooking Time: 35 Minutes
Ingredients:
- 2 cups heavy cream
- 1 cup milk
- 3/4 cup sugar
- 1 Tbs. vanilla extract
- 1 cup chocolate chips of your choice
- 2 tsps. cinnamon

Directions:
1. NOTE: Freeze your ice cream bowl for at least 24hrs prior to starting!
2. Place the milk and cream in a bowl, and mix them together until well combined. Use a whisk to mix in the sugar. Continue to whisk for about 4 minutes until the sugar dissolves. Then mix in the vanilla extract.
3. Pour the ingredients into your ice cream maker, and let it churn for 25 minutes. About 5 minutes before the ice cream is finished churning, add in the chocolate chips.
4. Serve immediately.

Thermomix Licorice Ice Cream

Servings: 12
Cooking Time: 30 Minutes
Ingredients:
- 3 cups heavy cream
- 2 cups whole milk
- ½ cup sugar
- A pinch of salt
- 6 egg yolks
- ½ teaspoon black food coloring
- ¼ cup soft licorice, chopped

Directions:
1. Add the cream, milk, sugar, and salt in a saucepan and heat over medium low flame. Simmer for 3 minutes or until the sugar dissolves. Remove from the stove.
2. In a bowl, whisk in the egg yolks. Drizzle ½ cup of the warm milk into the egg yolks while whisking constantly to form a smooth mixture. Whisk the egg mixture back into the pot. Add the black food coloring and licorice.
3. Turn on the heat to medium low and cook until the mixture starts to thicken. Constantly stir while cooking.
4. Turn off the heat and strain the mixture to remove lumps. Allow the milk to cool at room temperature. Place in the fridge to chill for 2 hours.
5. Turn on the Hamilton Beach and pour the mixture in. Churn for 15 minutes.
6. Transfer to an airtight container.

7. Place in the fridge to completely cool.

Nutrition Info: Calories per serving342 ; Protein 3g; Carbs 32g; Fat 22g Sugar 22g

Chocolate Chip Turmeric Peppermint Chip Ice Cream

Servings: 6
Cooking Time: 2 Hours 50 Minutes
Ingredients:

- 2 cups heavy cream
- 1 cup milk
- 3/4 cup sugar
- 1 teaspoon vanilla extract
- 1 teaspoon peppermint extract
- 1 cup semi-sweet chocolate chips
- 2 teaspoons turmeric

Directions:

1. NOTE: Freeze your ice cream bowl for at least 24hrs prior to starting!
2. Place the milk and cream in a bowl, and mix them together until well combined. Use a whisk to mix in the sugar. Continue to whisk for about 4 minutes until the sugar dissolves. Then mix in the vanilla, turmeric and peppermint extract.
3. Pour the ingredients into your ice cream maker, and let it churn for 25 minutes. About 5 minutes before the ice cream is finished churning, add in the chocolate chips.
4. Put the ice cream in an airtight container and place in the freezer for around 2 hours. Allow the ice cream to thaw for 15 minutes before serving.

Orange Cola Soft Serve Ice Cream

Servings: 6
Cooking Time: 55 Minutes
Ingredients:

- 2 cups heavy cream
- 1 cup milk
- 3/4 cup sugar
- 1 tbsp. orange extract
- 1 tbs. vanilla extract
- 3 cups coca cola (2, 12 ounce cans)

Directions:

1. NOTE: Freeze your ice cream bowl for at least 24hrs prior to starting!
2. Pour the coke into a large skillet, and heat it on high heat until it comes to a boil. Allow the coke to cook for about another 15 or 20 minutes, until the coke reduces down to 1 cup of liquid. Let the liquid cool.
3. Place the milk and cream in a bowl, and mix them together until well combined. Use a whisk to mix in the sugar. Continue to whisk for about 4 minutes until the sugar dissolves. Mix in the vanilla and orange extract, then the coca cola.
4. Pour the ingredients into your ice cream maker, and let it churn for 25 minutes.
5. Serve immediately.

Rhubarb Swirl Ice Cream

Servings: 10
Cooking Time: 45 Minutes
Ingredients:

- 4 stalks rhubarb, cut into ½ inch pieces
- 1 cup water
- ¾ cup sugar
- 1 cup ice cold whole milk
- ¾ cup sugar
- 1 ½ teaspoon pure vanilla extract
- A pinch of salt
- 2 cups cold heavy cream

Directions:

1. Place the rhubarb, water, and sugar in a saucepan and heat over high flame. Bring to a boil and cook while stirring constantly until the rhubarb will break down and turns into a jelly-like consistency. Set aside to cool.
2. Put ice water in a large mixing bowl. Place a small bowl on top of the large bowl with ice.
3. To the chilled small bowl, add the milk, sugar, vanilla, and salt. Whisk until well combined. Whisk in the heavy cream.
4. Turn on the Hamilton Beach and pour the mixture in. Freeze for 45 minutes.
5. Transfer into air-tight containers. Drizzle with the cooled rhubarb jelly and stir again.
6. Freeze overnight.

Nutrition Info: Calories per serving: 190; Protein: 3.5g; Carbs: 17.4g; Fat: 12.1g Sugar: 15.7g

Key Lime Ice Cream

Servings: 12
Cooking Time: 25 Minutes
Ingredients:
- 1 ½ cups ice cold whole milk, divided
- 2/3 cup sugar
- 1 ¼ cups ice cold heavy whipping cream
- ½ cup key lime juice, freshly squeezed
- 2 tablespoons light corn syrup
- ¼ tablespoon salt

Directions:
1. Put ice water in a large mixing bowl. Place a small bowl on top of the large bowl with ice.
2. Pour in the milk and sugar until well-combined. Add the cream and whip until well combined.
3. Stir in the rest of the ingredients while whipping constantly.
4. Turn on the Hamilton Beach and pour the mixture in. Freeze for 25 minutes.
5. Transfer into air-tight containers and freeze overnight.

Nutrition Info: Calories per serving: 96; Protein: 1.4g; Carbs: 11g; Fat: 5.6g Sugar: 10.2g

Tangerine Soda Ice Cream

Servings: 6
Cooking Time: 2 Hours 50 Minutes
Ingredients:
- 2 cups heavy cream
- 1 cup milk
- 3/4 cup sugar
- 1 teaspoon vanilla extract
- 20 ounces of your favorite orange soda
- orange extract (just a few drops)

Directions:
1. NOTE: Freeze your ice cream bowl for at least 24hrs prior to starting!
2. Place the milk and cream in a bowl, and mix them together until well combined. Use a whisk to mix in the sugar. Continue to whisk for about 4 minutes until the sugar dissolves. Then mix in the vanilla extract, orange soda and the few drops of orange extract.
3. Pour the ingredients into your ice cream maker, and let it churn for 25 minutes.
4. Put the ice cream in an airtight container and place in the freezer for around 2 hours. Allow the ice cream to thaw for 15 minutes before serving.

Honey Matcha Tea Extreme Ice Cream

Servings: 6
Cooking Time: 2 Hours 50 Minutes
Ingredients:
- 2 cups heavy cream
- 1 cup milk
- 3/4 cup sugar
- 1 teaspoon vanilla extract
- 1 tablespoon Matcha
- 3 tablespoons organic honey

Directions:
1. NOTE: Freeze your ice cream bowl for at least 24hrs prior to starting!
2. Place the milk and cream in a bowl, and mix them together until well combined. Use a whisk to mix in the sugar. Continue to whisk for about 4 minutes until the sugar dissolves. Then mix in the vanilla extract. Finally whisk in the Matcha until well mixed.
3. Pour the ingredients into your ice cream maker, and let it churn for 25 minutes.
4. Put the ice cream in an airtight container and place in the freezer for around 2 hours. Allow the ice cream to thaw for 15 minutes before serving.

Mocha Madness Ice Cream

Servings: 10
Cooking Time: 45 Minutes
Ingredients:
- 2 tablespoons unsweetened cocoa
- 2 tablespoons espresso powder
- 1 cup ice cold whole milk
- ¾ cup sugar
- 2 cups ice cold heavy cream
- 8 Oreo cookies, broken into small pieces

Directions:

1. Place cocoa, espresso powder, half of the milk and sugar in a pan. Bring to a simmer until everything dissolves. Turn off the heat and set aside in the fridge to cool.
2. Put ice water in a large mixing bowl. Place a small bowl on top of the large bowl with ice.
3. Pour in milk, sugar, espresso powder, and cocoa in the chilled bowl. Whisk until well combined.
4. Turn on the Hamilton Beach and pour the mixture in. Freeze for 45 minutes.
5. Transfer into air-tight containers and freeze overnight.

Nutrition Info: Calories per serving: 213; Protein: 4.2g; Carbs: 17.4g; Fat: 14.8g Sugar: 11.6g

Coffee Toffee Ice Cream

Servings: 10
Cooking Time: 45 Minutes
Ingredients:
- 1 ½ cups ice cold whole milk
- 1 1/8 cups granulated sugar
- 3 cups ice cold heavy cream
- 1 ½ tablespoons vanilla extract
- 4 tablespoons Instant Espresso Powder
- 12 ounces min chocolate bars, chopped

Directions:
1. Put ice water in a large mixing bowl. Place a small bowl on top of the large bowl with ice.
2. Place the milk and sugar in the bowl. Whisk to dissolve the sugar. Add the cream, vanilla extract, and espresso powder. Stir to combine everything.
3. Turn on the Hamilton Beach and pour the mixture in. Freeze for 45 minutes. Five minutes before the time, add the chopped chocolate bars.
4. Transfer into air-tight containers. Freeze overnight.

Nutrition Info: Calories per serving: 358; Protein: 6.6g; Carbs: 37.4g; Fat: 21.6g Sugar: 21g

Apricot Ice Cream

Servings: 10
Cooking Time: 45 Minutes
Ingredients:
- 1 ½ tablespoons lemon zest
- ½ cup apricot, mashed
- 1 cup sugar
- 1 ½ cups ice cold whole milk
- 1 ½ cups cold whipping cream

Directions:
1. Put ice water in a large mixing bowl. Place a small bowl on top of the large bowl with ice.
2. To the small bowl, whisk together the lemon zest, mashed apricot, sugar, and milk. Whisk until well combined.
3. Add the whipping cream then whisk again to incorporate all ingredients.
4. Turn on the Hamilton Beach and pour the mixture in. Freeze for 45 minutes.
5. Transfer into air-tight containers and freeze overnight.

Nutrition Info: Calories per serving: 143; Protein: 4.7g; Carbs: 16.5g; Fat: 6.8g Sugar: 14.2g

Chocolate Ice Cream

Servings: 10
Cooking Time: 25 Minutes
Ingredients:
- 1 cup whole milk
- ½ cup granulated sugar
- 8 ounces semi-sweet chocolate, chopped into small chunks
- 2 cups ice cold heavy cream
- 1 teaspoon pure vanilla extract

Directions:
1. Warm milk in a stovetop under low heat until the temperature reads at 175F. Stir in the sugar and chocolate until dissolved. Turn off the heat and set aside in the fridge to cool.
2. Put ice water in a large mixing bowl. Place a small bowl on top of the large bowl with ice. Pour the milk chocolate mixture into the small bowl and add heavy cream and vanilla.
3. Turn on the Hamilton Beach and pour the mixture in. Freeze for 25 minutes before transferring into an air-tight container.
4. Freeze inside the fridge overnight before serving.

Nutrition Info: Calories per serving:240 ; Protein: 2.1g; Carbs: 22.6g; Fat: 17g Sugar: 20.4g

Strawberry Matcha Custard Ice Cream

Servings: 10
Cooking Time: 30 Minutes
Ingredients:

- 3 cups heavy cream
- 1 cup milk
- ¾ cup sugar
- A pinch of salt
- 1 vanilla bean, scraped
- 6 egg yolks
- ½ cup chopped strawberries
- 3 tablespoons matcha or green tea powder

Directions:

1. Add the cream, milk, sugar, and salt in a saucepan and heat over medium low flame. Simmer for 3 minutes or until the sugar dissolves. Stir in the vanilla bean paste. Remove from the stove.
2. In a bowl, whisk in the egg yolks. Drizzle ½ cup of the warm milk into the egg yolks while whisking constantly to form a smooth mixture. Whisk the egg mixture back into the pot.
3. Turn on the heat to medium low and cook until the mixture starts to thicken. Constantly stir while cooking.
4. Turn off the heat and strain the mixture to remove lumps. Allow to cool at room temperature. Place in the fridge to chill for 2 hours.
5. Turn on the Hamilton Beach and pour the mixture in. Add the chopped strawberries. Churn for 15 minutes.
6. Transfer to an airtight container. Sprinkle with matcha powder on top.
7. Place in the fridge to completely cool.

Nutrition Info: Calories per serving:204 ; Protein: 3.2g; Carbs: 10.6g; Fat: 16.9g Sugar: 10g

Kiwi Lime Strawberry Ice Cream

Servings: 6
Cooking Time: 2 Hours 50 Minutes
Ingredients:

- 2 cups heavy cream
- 1 cup milk
- 3/4 cup sugar
- 1/2 teaspoon vanilla extract
- ½ teaspoon salt
- 1 kiwi, peeled
- 5 large strawberries chopped
- Juice of one and a half limes

Directions:

1. NOTE: Freeze your ice cream bowl for at least 24hrs prior to starting!
2. Puree the kiwi and strawberries in a food processor or blender.
3. Place the milk and cream in a bowl, and mix them together until well combined. Use a whisk to mix in the sugar and salt. Continue to whisk for about 4 minutes until the sugar and salt dissolves. Then mix in the vanilla extract, lime juice, and kiwi strawberry puree.
4. Pour the ingredients into your ice cream maker, and let it churn for 25 minutes.
5. Put the ice cream in an airtight container and place in the freezer for around 2 hours. Allow the ice cream to thaw for 15 minutes before serving.

Vegan Ice Cream

Servings: 12
Cooking Time: 45 Minutes
Ingredients:

- 2 13.5-ounce cans full-fat coconut milk
- ½ cup raw sugar
- 1 teaspoon vanilla extract
- 1 pinch xanthan gum
- ½ cup dark chocolate chips
- 1/3 cup roasted salted peanuts

Directions:

1. Pour in the coconut milk and sugar in a saucepan and whisk until well-combined. Add the vanilla and xanthan gum. Bring to a boil and whisk for 5 minutes.
2. Turn off the heat and allow to cool in the fridge for at least 6 hours.
3. Turn on the Hamilton Beach and pour the mixture in. Freeze for 45 minutes.
4. Add the chocolate chips and peanuts into the mixture 5 minutes before stopping the machine.
5. Transfer into air-tight containers and freeze overnight.

Nutrition Info: Calories per serving: 361; Protein: 4.1g; Carbs: 27.3g; Fat: 28.6g Sugar: 23.4g

Custard Chocolate Ice Cream

Servings: 10
Cooking Time: 30 Minutes
Ingredients:

- 1/3 cup unsweetened cocoa powder
- 2 cups heavy whipping cream
- 1 cup whole milk
- ¾ cup sugar
- 6 large egg yolks
- A pinch of salt
- 1 ½ teaspoons vanilla extract

Directions:
1. Add the coca powder, cream, milk and sugar in a saucepan and heat over medium low flame. Simmer for 3 minutes or until the sugar dissolves. Remove from the heat.
2. In a bowl, whisk in the egg yolks. Drizzle ½ cup of the warm milk into the egg yolks while whisking constantly to form a smooth mixture. Whisk the egg mixture back into the pot. Add the salt and vanilla.
3. Turn on the heat to medium low and cook until the mixture starts to thicken. Constantly stir while cooking.
4. Turn off the heat and strain the mixture to remove lumps. Allow the milk to cool at room temperature. Place in the fridge to chill for 2 hours.
5. Turn on the Hamilton Beach and pour the mixture in. Churn for 15 minutes.
6. Transfer to an airtight container.
7. Place in the fridge to completely cool.
Nutrition Info: Calories per serving: 175; Protein: 3.5g; Carbs: 13.4g; Fat: 12.7g Sugar: 11.3g

Graham Cracker Peanut Butter Cup Milkshake

Servings: 6
Cooking Time: 25 Minutes
Ingredients:

- 2 cups heavy cream
- 1 cup milk
- 3/4 cup sugar
- 1 tablespoon vanilla extract
- 1 1/2 cups chopped mini peanut butter cups
- ½ cup maple syrup
- 4 graham crackers

Directions:
1. NOTE: Freeze your ice cream bowl for at least 24hrs prior to starting!
2. Place the milk and cream in a bowl, and mix them together until well combined. Use a whisk to mix in the sugar. Continue to whisk for about 4 minutes until the sugar dissolves. Then mix in the vanilla extract.
3. Pour the ingredients into your ice cream maker, and let it churn for 10-15 minutes, until desired consistency is reached. About 5 minutes before the ice cream is done churning add the peanut butter cup and the graham crackers to your ice cream maker.
4. Serve immediately.

Crunchy Cinnamon Butterfinger Gelato

Servings: 4-6
Cooking Time: 2 Hours 35 Minutes
Ingredients:

- 1/2 cup heavy cream
- 2 cups milk
- 3/4 cup sugar
- 1 teaspoon vanilla extract
- 1 ½ cups chopped mini butterfinger bars
- 2 teaspoons ground cinnamon

Directions:
1. Refer to note at the beginning of the chapter about freezing bowl.
2. Place the milk and cream in a bowl, and mix them together until well combined. Use a whisk to mix in the sugar. Continue to whisk for about 4 minutes until the sugar dissolves. Then mix in the vanilla extract and cinnamon.
3. Pour the ingredients into your ice cream maker, and let it churn for 25 minutes. About 5 minutes before the ice cream is done churning add the butterfinger to your ice cream maker.
4. Put the gelato in an airtight container and place in the freezer for up to 2 hours, until desired consistency is reached.

Banana Custard Ice Cream

Servings: 8
Cooking Time: 30 Minutes
Ingredients:

- 2 cups heavy cream
- 2 cups half and half
- 5 tablespoons evaporated milk
- 1 ¼ cups granulated sugar
- ¼ teaspoon salt
- 4 egg yolks, beaten
- 1 cup mashed ripe bananas
- 2 tablespoons roasted peanuts, chopped

Directions:

1. Add the cream, half and half, milk, sugar, and salt in a saucepan and heat over medium low flame. Simmer for 3 minutes or until the sugar dissolves. Remove from the stove.
2. In a bowl, whisk in the egg yolks. Drizzle ½ cup of the warm milk into the egg yolks while whisking constantly to form a smooth mixture. Whisk the egg mixture back into the pot.
3. Turn on the heat to medium low and cook until the mixture starts to thicken. Constantly stir while cooking.
4. Turn off the heat and strain the mixture to remove lumps. Allow to cool at room temperature. Place in the fridge to chill for 2 hours.
5. Turn on the Hamilton Beach and pour the mixture in. Add the mashed bananas. Churn for 15 minutes.
6. Five minutes before the time ends, add the roasted peanuts.
7. Transfer to an airtight container.
8. Place in the fridge to completely cool.

Nutrition Info: Calories per serving: 298; Protein: 5.4g; Carbs: 35g; Fat:16.2 g Sugar: 26g

Chocolate Pistachio Ice Cream

Servings: 6
Cooking Time: 2 Hours 50 Minutes
Ingredients:

- 2 cups heavy cream
- 1 cup milk
- 3/4 cup sugar
- 1/4 teaspoon almond extract
- 1/2 cup chopped pistachios
- 1 cup semi-sweet chocolate chips

Directions:

1. NOTE: Freeze your ice cream bowl for at least 24hrs prior to starting!
2. Place the milk and cream in a bowl, and mix them together until well combined. Use a whisk to mix in the sugar. Continue to whisk for about 4 minutes until the sugar dissolves. Then mix in the almond extract.
3. Pour the ingredients into your ice cream maker, and let it churn for 25 minutes. About 5 minutes before the ice cream is finished churning, add in the pistachios and chocolate chips.
4. Put the ice cream in an airtight container and place in the freezer for around 2 hours. Allow the ice cream to thaw for 15 minutes before serving.

Butter Toffee Popcorn Soft Serve Ice Cream

Servings: 6
Cooking Time: 35 Minutes
Ingredients:

- 2 cups heavy cream
- 1 cup milk
- 3/4 cup sugar
- 1 Tbs. vanilla extract
- 2 cup butter toffee popcorn

Directions:

1. NOTE: Freeze your ice cream bowl for at least 24hrs prior to starting!
2. Place the milk and cream in a bowl, and mix them together until well combined. Use a whisk to mix in the sugar. Continue to whisk for about 4 minutes until the sugar dissolves. Mix in the vanilla extract. Place the mixture in a blender or food processor with 1 cup of the caramel corn, and puree.
3. Put the remaining caramel corn in a resealable plastic bag, and seal it. Crush the caramel corn using your hands, or a mallet.
4. Pour the ingredients into your ice cream maker, and let it churn for 25 minutes. About 5 minutes before the churning is finished add in the crushed caramel corn.
5. Serve immediately.

Cinnamon Blackberry Pineapple Ice Cream

Servings: 6
Cooking Time: 2 Hours 50 Minutes
Ingredients:
- 2 cups heavy cream
- 1 cup milk
- 3/4 cup sugar
- 1 teaspoon vanilla extract
- ½ cup pineapples
- ¼ cup of blackberries
- 1 tsp. cinnamon
- juice of 1/2 lemon

Directions:
1. NOTE: Freeze your ice cream bowl for at least 24hrs prior to starting!
2. Place the milk and cream in a bowl, and mix them together until well combined. Use a whisk to mix in the sugar. Continue to whisk for about 4 minutes until the sugar dissolves. Then mix in the vanilla extract, pineapples, blackberries lemon juice, and cinnamon.
3. Pour the ingredients into your ice cream maker, and let it churn for 25 minutes.
4. Put the ice cream in an airtight container and place in the freezer for around 2 hours. Allow the ice cream to thaw for 15 minutes before serving.

Bubble Gum Cola Soft Serve Ice Cream

Servings: 6
Cooking Time: 35 Minutes
Ingredients:
- 2 cups heavy cream
- 1 cup milk
- 3/4 cup sugar
- 1 Tbs. vanilla extract
- 1 gram bubble gum flavoring
- ½ cup mini gum balls
- ½ cup coca cola

Directions:
1. NOTE: Freeze your ice cream bowl for at least 24hrs prior to starting!
2. Place the milk and cream in a bowl, and mix them together until well combined. Use a whisk to mix in the sugar. Continue to whisk for about 4 minutes until the sugar dissolves. Mix in the vanilla extract, coca cola and then the bubble gum flavoring.
3. Pour the ingredients into your ice cream maker, and let it churn for 25 minutes. About 5 minutes before the churning is done add the gum balls to your ice cream maker.
4. Serve immediately.

Basic Custard Ice Cream With Sea Salt

Servings: 10
Cooking Time: 30 Minutes
Ingredients:
- 3 cups whole milk
- 1 cup sugar
- 8 egg yolks
- 1 teaspoon vanilla
- A pinch of coarse sea salt

Directions:
1. Add the milk and sugar in a saucepan and heat over medium low flame. Simmer for 3 minutes or until the sugar dissolves. Remove from the heat.
2. In a bowl, whisk in the egg yolks. Drizzle ½ cup of the warm milk into the egg yolks while whisking constantly to form a smooth mixture. Whisk the egg mixture back into the pot.
3. Turn on the heat to medium low and cook until the mixture starts to thicken. Constantly stir while cooking.
4. Turn off the heat and strain the mixture to remove lumps. Allow the milk to cool at room temperature. Place in the fridge to chill for 2 hours.
5. Turn on the Hamilton Beach and pour the mixture in. Churn for 15 minutes.
6. Transfer to an airtight container and sprinkle with sea salt on top.
7. Place in the fridge to completely cool.
Nutrition Info: Calories per serving: 50; Protein: 1.42g; Carbs: 6.7g; Fat: 2g Sugar: 5g

Fresh Strawberry Ice Cream

Servings: 10

Cooking Time: 25 Minutes

Ingredients:

- 1-pint strawberries, hulled and sliced
- 3 tablespoons lemon juice
- 1 cup white sugar, divided
- 1 cup ice cold whole milk
- 2 cups ice cold heavy cream
- 1 teaspoon vanilla extract

Directions:

1. Place half of the strawberries, lemon juice, and half of the sugar in a bowl. Macerate then strain to reserve the juice.
2. Chop the remaining strawberries. Set aside.
3. Put ice water in a large mixing bowl. Place a small bowl on top of the large bowl with ice.
4. Whisk together the whole milk, half of the sugar, heavy cream, and vanilla extract. Add the strawberry juice.
5. Turn on the Hamilton Beach and pour the mixture in. Freeze for 25 minutes. Five minutes before turning off the machine, add the chopped strawberries.
6. Transfer into air-tight containers and freeze overnight.

Nutrition Info: Calories per serving: 178; Protein: 3.5g; Carbs: 14.5g; Fat: 12.2g Sugar: 12.4g

Peach Ice Cream

Servings: 10
Cooking Time: 45 Minutes

Ingredients:

- 2 ripe peaches, peeled, pitted, and sliced
- 1 ½ cups ice cold whole milk
- 1 cup ice cold whipping cream
- 4 ounces cubed cream cheese, room temperature
- ½ cup sugar
- 2 tablespoons honey
- ½ teaspoon vanilla extract
- 1/8 teaspoon salt

Directions:

1. Put ice water in a large mixing bowl. Place a small bowl on top of the large bowl with ice.
2. Place the peaches in a blender and pulse until smooth.

3. Pour the peaches in the chilled bowl and add the milk, whipping cream, cream cheese, and sugar. Whisk until well combined and smooth. Add the honey, vanilla extract, and salt.
4. Turn on the Hamilton Beach and pour the mixture in. Freeze for 45 minutes.
5. Transfer into air-tight containers and freeze overnight.

Nutrition Info: Calories per serving:176 ; Protein: 5.6g; Carbs: 17.6 g; Fat: 9.7g Sugar: 14.2g

Tropical Coconut Banana Animal Cracker Sorbet

Servings: 4-8
Cooking Time: 2 Hours 40 Minutes

Ingredients:

- 3 peeled, mashed bananas
- 2-4 tablespoons honey to taste
- 1 1/2 cups light coconut milk
- 1 teaspoon vanilla extract
- 10 animal crackers

Directions:

1. NOTE: Freeze your ice cream bowl for at least 24hrs prior to starting!
2. Puree all ingredients in a food processor or blender. Taste, and add more honey if desired.
3. Pour the ingredients into your ice cream maker, and let it churn for 25-30 minutes. Mix in the animal crackers about 5 minutes before sorbet is complete.
4. Place in an airtight container for up to 2 hours, until desired consistency is reached.

Banana Pudding Ice Cream

Servings: 8
Cooking Time: 25 Minutes

Ingredients:

- 1 ½ cups half and half
- ½ cup packed brown sugar
- ½ cup white sugar
- 1/8 teaspoon salt
- 1 cup heavy whipping cream
- 1 ½ teaspoon vanilla extract
- 2 ripe bananas, mashed
- 1 cup crushed wafers, any brand

Directions:

1. Place the half and half, brown sugar, white sugar, and salt in a saucepan. Bring to a boil until the sugar dissolves. Turn off the heat and place in the fridge to cool.
2. Put ice water in a large mixing bowl. Place a small bowl on top of the large bowl with ice.
3. Place the cooled milk mixture in the bowl and add the whipping cream, vanilla extract, and bananas. Whisk to combine everything.
4. Turn on the Hamilton Beach and pour the mixture in. Freeze for 25 minutes. Five minutes before the time, add the wafers.
5. Transfer into air-tight containers. Freeze overnight.

Nutrition Info: Calories per serving:196 ; Protein: 2.6g; Carbs: 28.4g; Fat: 8.8g Sugar: 22.1g

Radical Root Beer Gelato

Servings: 4-6
Cooking Time: 2 Hours 50 Minutes
Ingredients:

- 1/2 cup heavy cream
- 2 cups milk
- 3/4 cup sugar
- 1 teaspoon vanilla extract
- 3 cups (2, 12 ounce cans) root beer

Directions:

1. Refer to note at the beginning of the chapter about freezing bowl.
2. Pour the root beer into a large skillet, and heat it on high heat until it comes to a boil. Allow the coke to cook for about another 15 or 20 minutes, until the root beer reduces down to 1 cup of liquid. Let the liquid cool.
3. Place the milk and cream in a bowl, and mix them together until well combined. Use a whisk to mix in the sugar. Continue to whisk for about 4 minutes until the sugar dissolves. Then mix in the vanilla extract and root beer reduction.
4. Pour the ingredients into your ice cream maker, and let it churn for 25 minutes. About 5 minutes before the ice cream is done churning add the chocolate to your ice cream maker.

5. Put the gelato in an airtight container and place in the freezer for up to 2 hours, until desired consistency is reached.

Eggless Pistachio Ice Cream

Servings: 10
Cooking Time: 45 Minutes
Ingredients:

- 1 cup ice cold whole milk
- 1 cup sugar
- 2 cups ice cold heavy cream
- ½ teaspoon vanilla extract
- 1 cup pistachio nuts, chopped

Directions:

1. Put ice water in a large mixing bowl. Place a small bowl on top of the large bowl with ice.
2. Place the milk and sugar in the bowl and whisk to dissolve the sugar. Add the cream and vanilla extract.
3. Turn on the Hamilton Beach and pour the mixture in. Freeze for 45 minutes. Five minutes before the time, add the pistachio nuts.
4. Transfer into air-tight containers. Freeze overnight.

Nutrition Info: Calories per serving:235 ; Protein: 5.8g; Carbs: 15.8g; Fat: 17.7g Sugar:11.5 g

Kiddo's Coca Cola Soft Serve Ice Cream

Servings: 6
Cooking Time: 55 Minutes
Ingredients:

- 2 cups heavy cream
- 1 cup milk
- 3/4 cup sugar
- 1 Tbs. vanilla extract
- 3 cups coca cola (2, 12 ounce cans)

Directions:

1. Refer to note at the beginning of the chapter about freezing bowl.
2. Pour the coke into a large skillet, and heat it on high heat until it comes to a boil. Allow the coke to cook for about another 15 or 20 minutes, until the coke reduces down to 1 cup of liquid. Let the liquid cool.

3.   Place the milk and cream in a bowl, and mix them together until well combined. Use a whisk to mix in the sugar. Continue to whisk for about 4 minutes until the sugar dissolves. Mix in the vanilla extract, and then the reduced coca cola.

4.   Pour the ingredients into your ice cream maker, and let it churn for 25 minutes.

5.   Serve immediately.

Dark Chocolate Cheery Custard Ice Cream

Servings: 12
Cooking Time: 30 Minutes
Ingredients:
- 1 cup whole milk
- 2 cups heavy cream
- 1 cup granulated sugar
- A pinch of salt
- 6 egg yolks
- 2 teaspoons vanilla extract
- ½ cup cherries, pitted and chopped
- ½ cup dark chocolate chips, shaved

Directions:
1.   Add the milk, cream, sugar, and salt in a saucepan and heat over medium low flame. Simmer for 3 minutes. Remove from the stove.

2.   In a bowl, whisk in the egg yolks. Drizzle ½ cup of the warm milk into the egg yolks while whisking constantly to form a smooth mixture. Whisk the egg mixture back into the pot. Add the vanilla extract.

3.   Turn on the heat to medium low and cook until the mixture starts to thicken. Constantly stir while cooking.

4.   Turn off the heat and strain the mixture to remove lumps. Allow to cool at room temperature. Place in the fridge to chill for 2 hours.

5.   Turn on the Hamilton Beach and pour the mixture in. Churn for 15 minutes.

6.   Before the churning time ends, add the cherries and chocolate shavings.

7.   Transfer to an airtight container.

8.   Place in the fridge to completely cool.

Nutrition Info: Calories per serving:196 ; Protein: 2.8g; Carbs: 18.1g; Fat: 12.6g Sugar: 14.8g

Turmeric Ice Cream

Servings: 10
Cooking Time: 30 Minutes
Ingredients:
- 3 cups whole milk
- 1 cup sugar
- 2 tablespoons turmeric powder
- 8 egg yolks
- A pinch of salt

Directions:
1.   Add the milk, sugar, and turmeric powder in a saucepan and heat over medium low flame. Simmer for 3 minutes or until the sugar dissolves. Remove from the heat.

2.   In a bowl, whisk in the egg yolks. Drizzle ½ cup of the warm milk into the egg yolks while whisking constantly to form a smooth mixture. Whisk the egg mixture back into the pot. Add the salt.

3.   Turn on the heat to medium low and cook until the mixture starts to thicken. Constantly stir while cooking.

4.   Turn off the heat and strain the mixture to remove lumps. Allow the milk to cool at room temperature. Place in the fridge to chill for 2 hours.

5.   Turn on the Hamilton Beach and pour the mixture in. Churn for 15 minutes.

6.   Transfer to an airtight container.

7.   Place in the fridge to completely cool.

Nutrition Info: Calories per serving:155 ; Protein: 5g; Carbs: 22g; Fat: 5g Sugar: 19g

Screamin' Sour Patch Kids Ice Cream

Servings: 6
Cooking Time: 2 Hours 50 Minutes
Ingredients:
- 2 cups heavy cream
- 1 cup milk
- 3/4 cup sugar
- 1 tablespoon vanilla extract
- 1 cups chopped sour patch kids

Directions:
1.   Refer to note at the beginning of the chapter about freezing bowl.

2.   Place the milk and cream in a bowl, and mix them together until well combined. Use a whisk to

mix in the sugar. Continue to whisk for about 4 minutes until the sugar dissolves. Then mix in the vanilla extract.

3. Pour the ingredients into your ice cream maker, and let it churn for 25 minutes. About 5 minutes before the ice cream is done churning add the sour patch kids to your ice cream maker.

4. Put the ice cream in an airtight container and place in the freezer for around 2 hours. Allow the ice cream to thaw for 15 minutes before serving.

My Delicious M&m Ice Cream

Servings: 6
Cooking Time: 2 Hours 50 Minutes
Ingredients:
- 2 cups heavy cream
- 1 cup milk
- 3/4 cup sugar
- 1 tablespoon vanilla extract
- 1 ½ cups M&Ms candy

Directions:
1. Refer to note at the beginning of the chapter about freezing bowl.

2. Place the milk and cream in a bowl, and mix them together until well combined. Use a whisk to mix in the sugar. Continue to whisk for about 4 minutes until the sugar dissolves. Then mix in the vanilla extract.

3. Pour the ingredients into your ice cream maker, and let it churn for 25 minutes. About 5 minutes before the ice cream is done churning add the M&Ms to your ice cream maker.

4. Put the ice cream in an airtight container and place in the freezer for around 2 hours. Allow the ice cream to thaw for 15 minutes before serving.

Pumpkin Custard Ice Cream

Servings: 6
Cooking Time: 30 Minutes
Ingredients:
- 2 cups heavy cream
- 2 cups milk
- ¼ cup granulated sugar
- ¾ cup brown sugar

- 1/8 teaspoon salt
- 3 egg yolk
- 1 teaspoon cinnamon
- ¼ teaspoon grated nutmeg
- 1/8 teaspoon ground cloves
- 1/8 teaspoon ground ginger
- 1 tablespoon vanilla extract
- 1 cup canned pumpkin, mashed

Directions:
1. Add the cream, milk, sugar, and salt in a saucepan and heat over medium low flame. Simmer for 3 minutes or until the sugar dissolves. Remove from the stove.

2. In a bowl, whisk in the egg yolks. Drizzle ½ cup of the warm milk into the egg yolks while whisking constantly to form a smooth mixture. Whisk the egg mixture back into the pot. Add the cinnamon, nutmeg, cloves, ginger, and vanilla.

3. Turn on the heat to medium low and cook until the mixture starts to thicken. Constantly stir while cooking.

4. Turn off the heat and strain the mixture to remove lumps. Allow the milk to cool at room temperature. Place in the fridge to chill for 2 hours.

5. Turn on the Hamilton Beach and pour the mixture in. Add the mashed pumpkin. Churn for 15 minutes.

6. Transfer to an airtight container.

7. Place in the fridge to completely cool.

Nutrition Info: Calories per serving:457 ; Protein: 10.7g; Carbs: 40g; Fat: 29g Sugar: 47g

Purple Taro Ice Cream

Servings: 10
Cooking Time: 1 Hour 15 Minutes
Ingredients:
- 1 cup purple taro, peeled and cubed
- 1 cup ice cold whole milk
- ¾ cup sugar
- 1 ½ cup ice cold heavy cream
- 2 tablespoons vanilla extract

Directions:
1. Place the purple taro in a saucepan and add enough water to cover the taro. Bring to a boil for 35 minutes or until soft. Drain to remove excess water.

Mash the purple taro using fork and remove big lumps. Set aside to cool.

2. Put ice water in a large mixing bowl. Place a small bowl on top of the large bowl with ice.

3. Place the milk and sugar in the bowl and stir to dissolve the sugar. Add the mashed and cooled taro in the mixture. Add the heavy cream and vanilla. Stir to combine.

4. Turn on the Hamilton Beach and pour the mixture in. Freeze for 45 minutes.

5. Transfer into air-tight containers.

6. Freeze overnight.

Nutrition Info: Calories per serving: 154; Protein: 3.3g; Carbs: 11.8 g; Fat: 9.9g Sugar: 8.3g

Blueberry Mint Soft Serve Ice Cream

Servings: 6

Cooking Time: 35 Minutes

Ingredients:

- 2 cups heavy cream
- 1 cup milk
- 3/4 cup sugar
- ½ cup blueberries
- 1 Tbs. vanilla extract
- 1 cup sliced peaches
- 1 hand full of mint leaves

Directions:

1. NOTE: Freeze your ice cream bowl for at least 24hrs prior to starting!

2. Puree the peaches and mint in a food processor or blender.

3. Place the milk and cream in a bowl, and mix them together until well combined. Use a whisk to mix in the sugar. Continue to whisk for about 4 minutes until the sugar dissolves. Then mix in the vanilla extract, blueberries and mint.

4. Pour the ingredients into your ice cream maker, and let it churn for 25 minutes.

5. Serve immediately.

California Mango Lime Soft Serve Ice Cream

Servings: 6

Cooking Time: 35 Minutes

Ingredients:

- 2 cups heavy cream
- 1 cup milk
- 3/4 cup sugar
- 1 Tbs. vanilla extract
- 1 cup pureed mango (about 2.5 mangos)
- Juice of 1 lime

Directions:

1. NOTE: Freeze your ice cream bowl for at least 24hrs prior to starting!

2. Puree the mangos with the lime juice in a food processor or blender.

3. Place the milk and cream in a bowl, and mix them together until well combined. Use a whisk to mix in the sugar. Continue to whisk for about 4 minutes until the sugar dissolves. Then mix in the vanilla extract. Then mix in the mango lime puree.

4. Pour the ingredients into your ice cream maker, and let it churn for 25 minutes.

5. Serve immediately.

Custard Cantaloupe Ice Cream

Servings: 10

Cooking Time: 30 Minutes

Ingredients:

- 3 cups whole milk
- 1 cup sugar
- 8 egg yolks
- A pinch of salt
- 1 cup cantaloupe, seeds removed and mashed

Directions:

1. Add the milk and sugar in a saucepan and heat over medium low flame. Simmer for 3 minutes or until the sugar dissolves. Remove from the heat.

2. In a bowl, whisk in the egg yolks. Drizzle ½ cup of the warm milk into the egg yolks while whisking constantly to form a smooth mixture. Whisk the egg mixture back into the pot. Add the salt.

3. Turn on the heat to medium low and cook until the mixture starts to thicken. Constantly stir while cooking.

4. Turn off the heat and strain the mixture to remove lumps. Allow the milk to cool at room temperature. Place in the fridge to chill for 2 hours.

5. Turn on the Hamilton Beach and pour the mixture in. Churn for 15 minutes.

6. Five minutes before the time ends, add the mashed cantaloupe.

7. Transfer to an airtight container.

8. Place in the fridge to completely cool.

Nutrition Info: Calories per serving:155 ; Protein: 4.5g; Carbs: 21.4g; Fat: 5.9g Sugar: 20.1g

Cookies And Cream Ice Cream

Servings: 10

Cooking Time: 30 Minutes

Ingredients:

- 2 cups heavy cream
- 1 cup whole milk
- ¾ cup sugar
- 2 teaspoons vanilla extract
- A pinch of salt
- 6 egg yolks
- 1 cup Oreo cookies, chopped

Directions:

1. Add the cream, milk, sugar, vanilla extract, and salt in a saucepan and heat over medium low flame. Simmer for 3 minutes or until the sugar dissolves. Remove from the stove.

2. In a bowl, whisk in the egg yolks. Drizzle ½ cup of the warm milk into the egg yolks while whisking constantly to form a smooth mixture. Whisk the egg mixture back into the pot.

3. Turn on the heat to medium low and cook until the mixture starts to thicken. Constantly stir while cooking.

4. Turn off the heat and strain the mixture to remove lumps. Allow to cool at room temperature. Place in the fridge to chill for 2 hours.

5. Turn on the Hamilton Beach and pour the mixture in. Churn for 15 minutes.

6. Five minutes before the time ends, add the chopped Oreo cookies.

7. Transfer to an airtight container.

8. Place in the fridge to completely cool.

Nutrition Info: Calories per serving:219 ; Protein: 4g; Carbs: 20 g; Fat: 13.9g Sugar: 15.5g

Red Velvet Milkshake

Servings: 6

Cooking Time: 25 Minutes

Ingredients:

- 2 cups heavy cream
- 1 cup milk
- 3/4 cup sugar
- 1 teaspoons vanilla extract
- 1 8 ounce package cream cheese, softened
- 1 tablespoon cocoa powder
- 1 tablespoon plus 1 teaspoon red food coloring

Directions:

1. Refer to note at the beginning of the chapter about freezing bowl.

2. Place the milk and cream in a bowl, and mix them together until well combined. Use a whisk to mix in the sugar. Continue to whisk for about 4 minutes until the sugar dissolves. Put all the ingredients in a blender and pulse for around 30 seconds until well mixed.

3. Pour the ingredients into your ice cream maker, and let it churn for 10-15 minutes, until desired consistency is reached.

4. Serve immediately.

Orange Creamsicle Ice Cream

Servings: 10

Cooking Time: 45 Minutes

Ingredients:

- ¼ cup water
- Zest from 1 orange
- ½ cup orange juice
- 1 tablespoon arrowroot powder
- 1 cup ice cold whole milk
- ¾ cup granulated sugar
- 2 cups heavy cream
- A pinch of salt

Directions:

1. Place half of the ¼ cup water orange zest, orange juice, and arrowroot powder in a saucepan. Stir to combine everything. Bring to a boil until the mixture thickens. Set aside to cool.

2. Put ice water in a large mixing bowl. Place a small bowl on top of the large bowl with ice.

3. Add the milk and sugar. Whisk until well combined. Stir in the cooled orange mixture and whisk until well incorporated and the lumps are dissolved. Add the rest of the ingredients.

4. Turn on the Hamilton Beach and pour the mixture in. Freeze for 45 minutes.

5. Transfer into air-tight containers.

6. Freeze overnight.

Nutrition Info: Calories per serving:164 ; Protein: 3.4g; Carbs: 11.1g; Fat: 12.1g Sugar: 9.1g

Blueberry Honey Cake Batter Soft Serve Ice Cream

Servings: 6
Cooking Time: 35 Minutes
Ingredients:

- 2 cups heavy cream
- 1 cup milk
- 3/4 cup sugar
- 1 Tbs. vanilla extract
- 2/3 cup cake mix
- ½ cup blueberries
- 2 tablespoons honey

Directions:

1. NOTE: Freeze your ice cream bowl for at least 24hrs prior to starting!

2. Place the milk and cream in a bowl, and mix them together until well combined. Use a whisk to mix in the sugar. Continue to whisk for about 4 minutes until the sugar dissolves. Mix in the vanilla extract, and then the 2/3 cup cake mix honey and blueberries.

3. Pour the ingredients into your ice cream maker, and let it churn for 25 minutes.

4. Serve immediately.

Butterfinger Cinnamon Crunch Gelato

Servings: 4-6
Cooking Time: 2 Hours 35 Minutes
Ingredients:

- 1/2 cup heavy cream
- 2 cups milk
- 3/4 cup sugar
- 1 teaspoon vanilla extract

- 1 ½ cups chopped mini Butterfinger bars
- 2 teaspoons ground cinnamon

Directions:

1. NOTE: Freeze your ice cream bowl for at least 24hrs prior to starting!

2. Place the milk and cream in a bowl, and mix them together until well combined. Use a whisk to mix in the sugar. Continue to whisk for about 4 minutes until the sugar dissolves. Then mix in the vanilla extract and cinnamon.

3. Pour the ingredients into your ice cream maker, and let it churn for 25 minutes. About 5 minutes before the ice cream is done churning add the Butterfinger to your ice cream maker.

4. Put the gelato in an airtight container and place in the freezer for up to 2 hours, until desired consistency is reached.

Crazy Cotton Candy Milkshake

Servings: 6
Cooking Time: 25 Minutes
Ingredients:

- 2 cups heavy cream
- 1 cup milk
- 3/4 cup sugar
- 1 teaspoon vanilla extract
- 1/2 cup cotton candy syrup
- 1 tablespoon plus 1 teaspoon pink or blue food coloring

Directions:

1. Refer to note at the beginning of the chapter about freezing bowl.

2. Place the milk and cream in a bowl, and mix them together until well combined. Use a whisk to mix in the sugar. Continue to whisk for about 4 minutes until the sugar dissolves. Then mix in the vanilla extract, syrup, and food coloring.

3. Pour the ingredients into your ice cream maker, and let it churn for 10-15 minutes, until desired consistency is reached.

4. Serve immediately.

Pralines And Cream Custard Ice Cream

Servings: 8

Cooking Time: 30 Minutes

Ingredients:

- 2 cups heavy cream
- 1 ½ cups half and half
- ¾ cup sugar
- 1 teaspoon vanilla extract
- ¼ teaspoon salt
- 4 egg yolks
- 1 cup caramel sauce
- 1 cup praline pecans

Directions:

1.   Add the cream, milk, sugar, vanilla extract, and salt in a saucepan and heat over medium low flame. Simmer for 3 minutes or until the sugar dissolves. Remove from the stove.

2.   In a bowl, whisk in the egg yolks. Drizzle ½ cup of the warm milk into the egg yolks while whisking constantly to form a smooth mixture. Whisk the egg mixture back into the pot.

3.   Turn on the heat to medium low and cook until the mixture starts to thicken. Constantly stir while cooking.

4.   Turn off the heat and strain the mixture to remove lumps. Allow to cool at room temperature. Place in the fridge to chill for 2 hours.

5.   Turn on the Hamilton Beach and pour the mixture in. Churn for 15 minutes.

6.   Five minutes before the time ends, add the caramel sauce and pecans.

7.   Transfer to an airtight container.

8.   Place in the fridge to completely cool.

Nutrition Info: Calories per serving: 474; Protein: 4g; Carbs: 46g; Fat: 32g Sugar: 24g

Peanut Butter Cup Milkshake

Servings: 6

Cooking Time: 25 Minutes

Ingredients:

- 2 cups heavy cream
- 1 cup milk
- 3/4 cup sugar
- 1 tablespoon vanilla extract
- 11/2 cups chopped mini peanut butter cups
- ½ cup maple syrup

Directions:

1.   Refer to note at the beginning of the chapter about freezing bowl.

2.   Place the milk and cream in a bowl, and mix them together until well combined. Use a whisk to mix in the sugar. Continue to whisk for about 4 minutes until the sugar dissolves. Then mix in the vanilla extract.

3.   Pour the ingredients into your ice cream maker, and let it churn for 10-15 minutes, until desired consistency is reached. About 5 minutes before the ice cream is done churning add the peanut butter cup to your ice cream maker.

4.   Serve immediately.

"cool" Cake Batter Soft Serve Ice Cream

Servings: 6

Cooking Time: 35 Minutes

Ingredients:

- 2 cups heavy cream
- 1 cup milk
- 3/4 cup sugar
- 1 Tbs. vanilla extract
- 2/3 cup cake mix

Directions:

1.   Refer to note at the beginning of the chapter about freezing bowl.

2.   Place the milk and cream in a bowl, and mix them together until well combined. Use a whisk to mix in the sugar. Continue to whisk for about 4 minutes until the sugar dissolves. Mix in the vanilla extract, and then the 2/3 cup cake mix.

3.   Pour the ingredients into your ice cream maker, and let it churn for 25 minutes.

4.   Serve immediately.

Peppermint Hibiscus Tea Ice Cream

Servings: 6

Cooking Time: 2 Hours 50 Minutes

Ingredients:

- 2 cups heavy cream
- 1 cup milk
- 3/4 cup sugar
- 1 teaspoon vanilla extract
- 2 tablespoons peppermint tea

- 2 tablespoons hibiscus tea

Directions:

1. NOTE: Freeze your ice cream bowl for at least 24hrs prior to starting!

2. Put the milk in a pan and bring it to a simmer. Add in the tea, take the pot off the heat, and allow to seep for 5 minutes. Discard the tea, and allow milk to cool.

3. Place the milk and cream in a bowl, and mix them together until well combined. Use a whisk to mix in the sugar. Continue to whisk for about 4 minutes until the sugar dissolves. Then mix in the vanilla extract.

4. Pour the ingredients into your ice cream maker, and let it churn for 25 minutes.

5. Put the ice cream in an airtight container and place in the freezer for around 2 hours. Allow the ice cream to thaw for 15 minutes before serving.

"georgia Peach" Maple Syrup Soft Serve Ice Cream

Servings: 6
Cooking Time: 35 Minutes

Ingredients:

- 2 cups heavy cream
- 1 cup milk
- 3/4 cup sugar
- 1 Tbs. vanilla extract
- 1 cup peaches
- ¼ cup maple syrup

Directions:

1. NOTE: Freeze your ice cream bowl for at least 24hrs prior to starting!

2. Puree the peaches in a food processor or blender.

3. Place the milk and cream in a bowl, and mix them together until well combined. Use a whisk to mix in the sugar. Continue to whisk for about 4 minutes until the sugar dissolves. Then mix in the vanilla extract. Then mix in the blueberries, and maple syrup.

4. Pour the ingredients into your ice cream maker, and let it churn for 25 minutes.

5. Serve immediately.

Circus Cotton Candy Milkshake

Servings: 6
Cooking Time: 25 Minutes

Ingredients:

- 2 cups heavy cream
- 1 cup milk
- 3/4 cup sugar
- 1 teaspoon vanilla extract
- 1/2 cup cotton candy syrup
- 1 tablespoon plus 1 teaspoon pink or blue food coloring

Directions:

1. NOTE: Freeze your ice cream bowl for at least 24hrs prior to starting!

2. Place the milk and cream in a bowl, and mix them together until well combined. Use a whisk to mix in the sugar. Continue to whisk for about 4 minutes until the sugar dissolves. Then mix in the vanilla extract, syrup, and food coloring.

3. Pour the ingredients into your ice cream maker, and let it churn for 10-15 minutes, until desired consistency is reached.

4. Serve immediately.

Green Apple Musketeer Gelato

Servings: 4-6
Cooking Time: 2 Hours 35 Minutes

Ingredients:

- 1/2 cup heavy cream
- 2 cups milk
- 3/4 cup sugar
- 1 tablespoon vanilla extract
- 1 ½ cups chopped mini Musketeers bars
- ¼ cup green apples

Directions:

1. NOTE: Freeze your ice cream bowl for at least 24hrs prior to starting!

2. Place the milk and cream in a bowl, and mix them together until well combined. Use a whisk to mix in the sugar. Continue to whisk for about 4 minutes until the sugar dissolves. Then mix in the vanilla extract.

3. Pour the ingredients into your ice cream maker, and let it churn for 25 minutes. About 5 minutes before the ice cream is done churning add the three

musketeers and green apples to your ice cream maker.

4.   Put the gelato in an airtight container and place in the freezer for up to 2 hours, until desired consistency is reached.

Dr. Pepper Ice Cream

Servings: 6
Cooking Time: 2 Hours 50 Minutes
Ingredients:
- 2 cups heavy cream
- 1 cup milk
- 3/4 cup sugar
- 1 tablespoon vanilla extract
- 3 cups (2, 12 ounce cans) dr. pepper

Directions:
1.   Refer to note at the beginning of the chapter about freezing bowl.
2.   Pour the dr. pepper into a large skillet, and heat it on high heat until it comes to a boil. Allow the coke to cook for about another 15 or 20 minutes, until the root beer reduces down to 1 cup of liquid. Let the liquid cool.
3.   Place the milk and cream in a bowl, and mix them together until well combined. Use a whisk to mix in the sugar. Continue to whisk for about 4 minutes until the sugar dissolves. Then mix in the vanilla extract and dr. pepper reduction.
4.   Pour the ingredients into your ice cream maker, and let it churn for 25 minutes. \
5.   Put the ice cream in an airtight container and place in the freezer for around 2 hours. Allow the ice cream to thaw for 15 minutes before serving.

"crispy" Caramel Graham Cracker Ice Cream

Servings: 6
Cooking Time: 2 Hours 50 Minutes
Ingredients:
- 2 cups heavy cream
- 1 cup milk
- 3/4 cup sugar
- 1 tablespoon vanilla extract
- 1 ½ cups chopped mini Kit Kats

- 2 oz. caramel

Directions:
1.   NOTE: Freeze your ice cream bowl for at least 24hrs prior to starting!
2.   Place the milk and cream in a bowl, and mix them together until well combined. Use a whisk to mix in the sugar. Continue to whisk for about 4 minutes until the sugar dissolves. Then mix in the vanilla extract.
3.   Warm up the caramel to add to the ice cream maker towards the end of the process.
4.   Pour the ingredients into your ice cream maker, and let it churn for 25 minutes. About 5 minutes before the ice cream is done churning add the graham crackers and caramel to the machine.
5.   Put the ice cream in an airtight container and place in the freezer for around 2 hours. Allow the ice cream to thaw for 15 minutes before serving.

Pineapple Ice Cream

Servings: 6
Cooking Time: 45 Minutes
Ingredients:
- 1 ½ cup pineapple juice
- 1 can crushed pineapple
- ½ cup heavy whipping cream

Directions:
1.   Put ice water in a large mixing bowl. Place a small bowl on top of the large bowl with ice.
2.   Place all ingredients in the small bowl. Whisk until well combined.
3.   Turn on the Hamilton Beach and pour the mixture in. Freeze for 45 minutes.
4.   Transfer into air-tight containers.
5.   Freeze overnight.

Nutrition Info: Calories per serving: 136; Protein: 1g; Carbs: 26g; Fat: 3.8g Sugar: 24g

Cinnamon Ice Cream

Servings: 10
Cooking Time: 45 Minutes
Ingredients:
- 2 cups heavy cream
- 1 cup half and half

- ½ cup sugar
- ¼ cup brown sugar
- 1 teaspoon vanilla extract
- 1 tablespoon cinnamon
- A pinch of salt

Directions:

1. Put ice water in a large mixing bowl. Place a small bowl on top of the large bowl with ice.
2. Pour all ingredients in the bowl. Whisk until well-combined.
3. Turn on the Hamilton Beach and pour the mixture in. Freeze for 45 minutes.
4. Transfer into air-tight containers. Freeze overnight.

Nutrition Info: Calories per serving: 140; Protein: 1.1g; Carbs: 13.8 g; Fat: 9.2g Sugar: 12.1g

Vanilla Frozen Custard

Servings: 6
Cooking Time: 30 Minutes
Ingredients:

- 2 cups heavy cream
- 1 cup whole milk
- 2/3 cup granulated sugar
- A pinch of salt
- 6 large egg yolks
- 2 teaspoons vanilla extract

Directions:

1. Add the cream, milk, sugar, and salt in a saucepan and heat over medium low flame. Simmer for 3 minutes or until the sugar dissolves.
2. Remove from the heat.
3. In a bowl, whisk in the egg yolks. Drizzle ½ cup of the warm milk into the egg yolks while whisking constantly to form a smooth mixture. Whisk the egg mixture back into the pot and add vanilla.
4. Turn on the heat to medium low and cook until the mixture starts to thicken. Constantly stir while cooking.
5. Turn off the heat and strain the mixture to remove lumps. Allow the milk to cool at room temperature. Place in the fridge to chill for 2 hours.
6. Turn on the Hamilton Beach and pour the mixture in. Churn for 15 minutes.

7. Transfer to an airtight container and place in the fridge to completely cool.

Nutrition Info: Calories per serving: 443; Protein: 5g; Carbs: 27 g; Fat: 35g Sugar: 24g

Chicago Style Cookies-n-cream Soft Serve Ice Cream

Servings: 6
Cooking Time: 35 Minutes
Ingredients:

- 2 cups heavy cream
- 1 cup milk
- 3/4 cup sugar
- 1 Tbs. vanilla extract
- 20 chocolate sandwich cookies

Directions:

1. NOTE: Freeze your ice cream bowl for at least 24hrs prior to starting!
2. Place the milk and cream in a bowl, and mix them together until well combined. Use a whisk to mix in the sugar. Continue to whisk for about 4 minutes until the sugar dissolves. Then mix in the vanilla extract.
3. Place the sandwich cookies in a food processor, and process until the cookies are no bigger than chocolate chips. If you don't have a food processor place the cookies in a large resealable plastic bag, and seal it shut. Use your hands, a mallet, or a rolling pin to crush the cookies.
4. Pour the ingredients into your ice cream maker, and let it churn for 25 minutes. About 5 minutes before the ice cream is finished churning, add in the chocolate sandwich cookies.
5. Serve immediately.

Cherry Blueberry Lime Soda Frozen Yogurt

Servings: 1 Quart
Cooking Time: 2 Hours 50 Minutes
Ingredients:

- 1 quart container full-fat plain yogurt
- ¼ teaspoon salt
- 1 cup sugar
- ½ lime (peeled and cut up fine)

- 1/2 cup blueberries
- 1 teaspoon vanilla extract
- 3 cups (2, 12 ounce cans) cherry soda

Directions:

1. NOTE: Freeze your ice cream bowl for at least 24hrs prior to starting!
2. Pour the cherry soda into a large skillet, and heat it on high heat until it comes to a boil. Allow the coke to cook for about another 15 or 20 minutes, until the root beer reduces down to 1 cup of liquid. Let the liquid cool.
3. Place the yogurt in a bowl. Use a whisk to mix in the sugar and salt. Continue to whisk for about 4 minutes until the sugar dissolves. Then mix in the vanilla extract, blueberries, lime and reduced cherry soda.
4. Pour the ingredients into your ice cream maker, and let it churn for 25 minutes.
5. Put the frozen yogurt in an airtight container and place in the freezer for at least 2 hours, until desired consistency is reached.

Double Bubble Gum Soft Serve Ice Cream

Servings: 6

Cooking Time: 35 Minutes

Ingredients:

- 2 cups heavy cream
- 1 cup milk
- 3/4 cup sugar
- 1 Tbs. vanilla extract
- 1 dram bubble gum flavoring
- ½ cup mini gum balls

Directions:

1. Refer to note at the beginning of the chapter about freezing bowl.
2. Place the milk and cream in a bowl, and mix them together until well combined. Use a whisk to mix in the sugar. Continue to whisk for about 4 minutes until the sugar dissolves. Mix in the vanilla extract, and then the bubble gum flavoring.
3. Pour the ingredients into your ice cream maker, and let it churn for 25 minutes. About 5 minutes before the churning is done add the gum balls to your ice cream maker.
4. Serve immediately.

Mocha Ice Cream

Servings: 10

Cooking Time: 25 Minutes

Ingredients:

- 1 cup ice cold whole milk
- ¼ cup granulated sugar
- 2 cups heavy cream
- 1 teaspoon vanilla extract
- 2 tablespoons instant coffee, dissolved in 3 tablespoons hot water

Directions:

1. Put ice water in a large mixing bowl. Place a small bowl on top of the large bowl with ice.
2. Pour the milk in the small bowl and add the sugar. Whisk until well-combined and the sugar dissolves. Add the rest of the ingredients and whisk.
3. Turn on the Hamilton Beach and pour the mixture in. Freeze for 25 minutes.
4. Transfer into air-tight containers and freeze overnight.

Nutrition Info: Calories per serving:139 ; Protein: 3.4g; Carbs: 4.4g; Fat: 12.1g Sugar: 3.2g

Red Velvet Raspberry Milkshake

Servings: 6

Cooking Time: 25 Minutes

Ingredients:

- 2 cups heavy cream
- 1 cup milk
- 3/4 cup sugar
- 1 teaspoons vanilla extract
- 1 - 8-ounce package cream cheese, softened
- 1 tablespoon cocoa powder
- 1 tablespoon & 1 teaspoon red food coloring
- ¼ cup raspberries

Directions:

1. NOTE: Freeze your ice cream bowl for at least 24hrs prior to starting!
2. Place the milk and cream in a bowl, and mix them together until well combined. Use a whisk to mix in the sugar. Continue to whisk for about 4 minutes until the sugar dissolves. Put all the

ingredients in a blender and pulse for around 30 seconds until well mixed.

3. Pour the ingredients into your ice cream maker, and let it churn for 10-15 minutes, until desired consistency is reached.

4. Serve immediately.

Sour Patch Chocolate Ice Cream

Servings: 6

Cooking Time: 2 Hours 50 Minutes

Ingredients:

- 2 cups heavy cream
- 1 cup milk
- 3/4 cup sugar
- 1 tablespoon vanilla extract
- 1 cups chopped sour patch
- ½ cup chocolate (chopped fine)

Directions:

1. NOTE: Freeze your ice cream bowl for at least 24hrs prior to starting!

2. Place the milk and cream in a bowl, and mix them together until well combined. Use a whisk to mix in the sugar. Continue to whisk for about 4 minutes until the sugar dissolves. Then mix in the vanilla extract.

3. Pour the ingredients into your ice cream maker, and let it churn for 25 minutes. About 5 minutes before the ice cream is done churning add the sour patch and chocolate to your ice cream maker.

4. Put the ice cream in an airtight container and place in the freezer for around 2 hours. Allow the ice cream to thaw for 15 minutes before serving.

Custard Cream Gelato

Servings: 20

Cooking Time: 30 Minutes

Ingredients:

- 6 cups whole milk
- 1 1/3 cups sugar
- 12 egg yolks
- 1 medium lemon juice

Directions:

1. Add the milk and sugar in a saucepan and heat over medium low flame. Simmer for 3 minutes or until the sugar dissolves. Remove from the stove.

2. In a bowl, whisk in the egg yolks. Drizzle ½ cup of the warm milk into the egg yolks while whisking constantly to form a smooth mixture. Whisk the egg mixture back into the pot. Add the lemon juice while stirring constantly.

3. Turn on the heat to medium low and cook until the mixture starts to thicken. Constantly stir while cooking.

4. Turn off the heat and strain the mixture to remove lumps. Allow the milk to cool at room temperature. Place in the fridge to chill for 2 hours.

5. Turn on the Hamilton Beach and pour the mixture in. Churn for 15 minutes.

6. Transfer to an airtight container.

7. Place in the fridge to completely cool.

Nutrition Info: Calories per serving:125 ; Protein: 3.8g; Carbs: 16.6g; Fat: 4.9g Sugar: 16g

Dr. Pepper Cherry Lime Ice Cream

Servings: 6

Cooking Time: 2 Hours 50 Minutes

Ingredients:

- 2 cups heavy cream
- 1 cup milk
- 3/4 cup sugar
- 1 tablespoon vanilla extract
- 3 cups (2, 12 ounce cans) Dr. Pepper
- ½ cup mashed up cherries
- 1 tablespoon lime juice

Directions:

1. NOTE: Freeze your ice cream bowl for at least 24hrs prior to starting!

2. Pour the dr. pepper into a large skillet, and heat it on high heat until it comes to a boil. Allow the coke to cook for about another 15 or 20 minutes, until the root beer reduces down to 1 cup of liquid. Let the liquid cool.

3. Place the milk and cream in a bowl, and mix them together until well combined. Use a whisk to mix in the sugar. Continue to whisk for about 4 minutes until the sugar dissolves. Then mix in the

vanilla extract, lime juice Dr. pepper reduction and cherries.

4. Pour the ingredients into your ice cream maker, and let it churn for 25 minutes. \

5. Put the ice cream in an airtight container and place in the freezer for around 2 hours. Allow the ice cream to thaw for 15 minutes before serving.

Chilled Cherry Soda Frozen Yogurt

Servings: 1 Quart
Cooking Time: 2 Hours 50 Minutes
Ingredients:
- 1 quart container full-fat plain yogurt
- ¼ teaspoon salt
- 1 cup sugar
- 1 teaspoon vanilla extract
- 3 cups (2, 12 ounce cans) cherry soda

Directions:
1. Refer to note at the beginning of the chapter about freezing bowl.

2. Pour the cherry soda into a large skillet, and heat it on high heat until it comes to a boil. Allow the coke to cook for about another 15 or 20 minutes, until the root beer reduces down to 1 cup of liquid. Let the liquid cool.

3. Place the yogurt in a bowl. Use a whisk to mix in the sugar and salt. Continue to whisk for about 4 minutes until the sugar dissolves. Then mix in the vanilla extract, and reduced cherry soda.

4. Pour the ingredients into your ice cream maker, and let it churn for 25 minutes.

5. Put the frozen yogurt in an airtight container and place in the freezer for at least 2 hours, until desired consistency is reached.

Caramel Corn Soft Serve Ice Cream

Servings: 6
Cooking Time: 35 Minutes
Ingredients:
- 2 cups heavy cream
- 1 cup milk
- 3/4 cup sugar
- 1 Tbs. vanilla extract
- 2 cup caramel corn

Directions:
1. Refer to note at the beginning of the chapter about freezing bowl.

2. Place the milk and cream in a bowl, and mix them together until well combined. Use a whisk to mix in the sugar. Continue to whisk for about 4 minutes until the sugar dissolves. Mix in the vanilla extract. Place the mixture in a blender or food processor with 1 cup of the caramel corn, and puree.

3. Put the remaining caramel corn in a resealable plastic bag, and seal it. Crush the caramel corn using your hands, or a mallet.

4. Pour the ingredients into your ice cream maker, and let it churn for 25 minutes. About 5 minutes before the churning is finished add in the crushed caramel corn.

5. Serve immediately.

Nutella Ice Cream

Servings: 10
Cooking Time: 30 Minutes
Ingredients:
- 2 cups heavy cream
- 1 cup whole milk
- 2/3 cup granulated sugar
- 1 teaspoon salt
- 6 egg yolks
- ½ cup Nutella
- 1 teaspoon vanilla extract

Directions:
1. Add the cream, milk, sugar, and salt in a saucepan and heat over medium low flame. Simmer for 3 minutes. Remove from the stove.

2. In a bowl, whisk in the egg yolks. Drizzle ½ cup of the warm milk into the egg yolks while whisking constantly to form a smooth mixture. Whisk the egg mixture back into the pot.

3. Turn on the heat to medium low and cook until the mixture starts to thicken. Constantly stir while cooking. Add Nutella and vanilla.

4. Turn off the heat and strain the mixture to remove lumps. Allow to cool at room temperature. Place in the fridge to chill for 2 hours.

5. Turn on the Hamilton Beach and pour the mixture in. Churn for 15 minutes.

6. Transfer to an airtight container.

7. Place in the fridge to completely cool.

Nutrition Info: Calories per serving: 219; Protein: 3.4g; Carbs: 17.4g; Fat: 15.3g Sugar: 15.8g

Honey Ice Cream

Servings: 12

Cooking Time: 30 Minutes

Ingredients:

- 1 ½ cups heavy cream
- 1 ½ cups whole milk
- ½ cup honey
- ½ teaspoon salt
- 4 large egg yolks
- 1 ½ teaspoon vanilla extract

Directions:

1. Add the cream, milk, honey, and salt in a saucepan and heat over medium low flame. Simmer for 3 minutes or until the sugar dissolves.

2. In a bowl, whisk in the egg yolks. Drizzle ½ cup of the warm milk into the egg yolks while whisking constantly to form a smooth mixture. Whisk the egg mixture back into the pot.

3. Turn on the heat to medium low and cook until the mixture starts to thicken. Constantly stir while cooking.

4. Turn off the heat and strain the mixture to remove lumps. Allow the milk to cool at room temperature. Place in the fridge to chill for 2 hours.

5. Turn on the Hamilton Beach and pour the mixture in. Churn for 15 minutes.

6. Transfer to an airtight container.

7. Place in the fridge to completely cool.

Nutrition Info: Calories per serving:142 ; Protein: 2.2g; Carbs: 16.3g; Fat: 8g Sugar: 16g

Orange Almond Apricot Ice Cream

Servings: 6

Cooking Time: 2 Hours 50 Minutes

Ingredients:

- 2 cups heavy cream
- 1 cup milk
- 3/4 cup sugar
- 1 teaspoon vanilla extract
- 1 cup sliced apricots
- ½ cup chopped almonds
- orange extract (just a few drops will do)

Directions:

1. ❯NOTE: Freeze your ice cream bowl for at least 24hrs prior to starting!

2. Puree the apricots in a food processor or blender.

3. Place the milk and cream in a bowl, and mix them together until well combined. Use a whisk to mix in the sugar. Continue to whisk for about 4 minutes until the sugar dissolves. Then mix in the vanilla extract, and apricot puree.

4. Pour the ingredients into your ice cream maker, and let it churn for 25 minutes. About 5 minutes before the ice cream is finished churning, add in the almonds and orange extract.

5. Put the ice cream in an airtight container and place in the freezer for around 2 hours. Allow the ice cream to thaw for 15 minutes before serving.

All-american Double Vanilla Soft-serve Ice Cream

Servings: 6

Cooking Time: 35 Minutes

Ingredients:

- 2 cups heavy cream
- 1 cup milk
- 3/4 cup sugar
- 2 Tbs. vanilla extract

Directions:

1. NOTE: Freeze your ice cream bowl for at least 24hrs prior to starting!

2. Place the milk and cream in a bowl, and mix them together until well combined. Use a whisk to mix in the sugar. Continue to whisk for about 4 minutes until the sugar dissolves. Then mix in the vanilla extract.

3. Pour the ingredients into your ice cream maker, and let it churn for 25 minutes.

4. Serve immediately.

Gummy Worm Cotton Candy Ice Cream

Servings: 6

Cooking Time: 2 Hours 50 Minutes

Ingredients:

- 2 cups heavy cream
- 1 cup milk
- 3/4 cup sugar
- 1 tablespoon vanilla extract
- 1 tablespoon cotton candy extract
- 1 ½ cups gummy worm candy

Directions:

1. NOTE: Freeze your ice cream bowl for at least 24hrs prior to starting!
2. Place the milk and cream in a bowl, and mix them together until well combined. Use a whisk to mix in the sugar. Continue to whisk for about 4 minutes until the sugar dissolves. Then mix in the vanilla extract.
3. Pour the ingredients into your ice cream maker, and let it churn for 25 minutes. About 5 minutes before the ice cream is done churning add the M&Ms to your ice cream maker.
4. Put the ice cream in an airtight container and place in the freezer for around 2 hours. Allow the ice cream to thaw for 15 minutes before serving.

"give Me More" S'mores Frozen Yogurt

Servings: 1 Quart
Cooking Time: 2 Hours 35 Minutes

Ingredients:

- 1 quart container full-fat plain yogurt
- ¼ teaspoon salt
- 1 cup sugar
- 1 teaspoon vanilla extract
- 3 large graham crackers
- 4 ounces chopped semi-sweet chocolate
- ½ cup mini marshmallows

Directions:

1. Refer to note at the beginning of the chapter about freezing bowl.
2. Place the yogurt in a bowl. Use a whisk to mix in the sugar and salt. Continue to whisk for about 4 minutes until the sugar dissolves. Then mix in the vanilla extract.
3. Place the graham crackers in a food processor, and process until the crackers are no bigger than chocolate chips. If you don't have a food processor

place the crackers in a large resealable plastic bag, and seal it shut. Use your hands, a mallet, or a rolling pin to crush the cookies.
4. Pour the ingredients into your ice cream maker, and let it churn for 25 minutes. About 5 minutes before the ice cream is done churning add the chocolate, graham crackers, and marshmallows to your ice cream maker.
5. Put the frozen yogurt in an airtight container and place in the freezer for at least 2 hours, until desired consistency is reached.

Barbados Custard Ice Cream

Servings: 12
Cooking Time: 30 Minutes

Ingredients:

- 2 cups whole milk
- ½ cup sugar
- ¼ cup light brown sugar
- A pinch of salt
- 1 vanilla pod, scraped
- 6 egg yolks
- ½ cup crème fraiche
- 1 tablespoon dark rum

Directions:

1. Add the milk, sugar, and salt in a saucepan and heat over medium low flame. Simmer for 3 minutes or until the sugar dissolves. Remove from the stove.
2. In a bowl, whisk in the egg yolks. Drizzle ½ cup of the warm milk into the egg yolks while whisking constantly to form a smooth mixture. Whisk the egg mixture back into the pot. Add the vanilla, crème fraiche, and rum.
3. Turn on the heat to medium low and cook until the mixture starts to thicken. Constantly stir while cooking.
4. Turn off the heat and strain the mixture to remove lumps. Allow to cool at room temperature. Place in the fridge to chill for 2 hours.
5. Turn on the Hamilton Beach and pour the mixture in. Churn for 15 minutes.
6. Transfer to an airtight container.
7. Place in the fridge to completely cool.

Nutrition Info: Calories per serving: 103; Protein: 2.7g; Carbs: 10.2g; Fat: 5.5g Sugar: 9.6g

Rocky Road Frozen Custard Ice Cream

Servings: 12
Cooking Time: 30 Minutes
Ingredients:
- 1 cup whole milk
- 2 cups heavy cream
- ¾ cup sugar
- ½ teaspoon salt
- 2 tablespoons unsweetened cocoa powder
- ½ teaspoon ground cinnamon
- 3 egg yolks
- 2 ounces chocolate bar, chopped
- 1 cup mini marshmallows
- ½ cup toasted pecans

Directions:
1.   Add the milk, cream, sugar, and salt in a saucepan and heat over medium low flame. Simmer for 3 minutes or until the sugar dissolves. Add the cocoa powder and cinnamon. Stir for another minute. Remove from the heat.
2.   In a bowl, whisk in the egg yolks. Drizzle ½ cup of the warm milk into the egg yolks while whisking constantly to form a smooth mixture. Whisk the egg mixture back into the pot.
3.   Turn on the heat to medium low and cook until the mixture starts to thicken. Constantly stir while cooking.
4.   Turn off the heat and strain the mixture to remove lumps. Allow the milk to cool at room temperature. Place in the fridge to chill for 2 hours.
5.   Turn on the Hamilton Beach and pour the mixture in. Churn for 15 minutes.
6.   Five minutes before the time ends, add the chopped chocolate, marshmallows, and pecans.
7.   Transfer to an airtight container.
8.   Place in the fridge to completely cool.
Nutrition Info: Calories per serving: 189; Protein: 2.6g; Carbs: 13.8g; Fat: 14.4g Sugar: 11.3g

Blackberry Ice Cream

Servings: 10
Cooking Time: 45 Minutes
Ingredients:
- 1 ½ cups blackberries, frozen or fresh
- ¾ cup ice cold whole milk
- ½ cup sugar
- A pinch of salt
- 1 ½ cup heavy cream, ice cold
- 1 ½ teaspoon vanilla

Directions:
1.   Clean the blackberries by removing the stem and seeds. Mash to release the juice and pass through a sieve. Save the juice and set aside.
2.   Put ice water in a large mixing bowl. Place a small bowl on top of the large bowl with ice.
3.   Place the whole milk, sugar, and salt. Whisk to combine everything. Add the cream, vanilla, and blackberry juice. Stir to combined.
4.   Turn on the Hamilton Beach and pour the mixture in. Freeze for 45 minutes.
5.   Transfer into air-tight containers.
6.   Freeze overnight.
Nutrition Info: Calories per serving: 151; Protein: 3g; Carbs: 15g; Fat: 9.1g Sugar: 13.1g

Three Musketeer Gelato

Servings: 4-6
Cooking Time: 2 Hours 35 Minutes
Ingredients:
- 1/2 cup heavy cream
- 2 cups milk
- 3/4 cup sugar
- 1 tablespoon vanilla extract
- 1 ½ cups chopped mini three musketeers bars

Directions:
1.   Refer to note at the beginning of the chapter about freezing bowl.
2.   Place the milk and cream in a bowl, and mix them together until well combined. Use a whisk to mix in the sugar. Continue to whisk for about 4 minutes until the sugar dissolves. Then mix in the vanilla extract.
3.   Pour the ingredients into your ice cream maker, and let it churn for 25 minutes. About 5 minutes before the ice cream is done churning add the three musketeers to your ice cream maker.

4. Put the gelato in an airtight container and place in the freezer for up to 2 hours, until desired consistency is reached.

Classic Root Beer Lemon Gelato

Servings: 4-6
Cooking Time: 2 Hours 50 Minutes
Ingredients:
- 1/2 cup heavy cream
- 2 cups milk
- 3/4 cup sugar
- 1 teaspoon vanilla extract
- 3 cups (2, 12 ounce cans) root beer
- 2 tablespoons lemon juice

Directions:
1. NOTE: Freeze your ice cream bowl for at least 24hrs prior to starting!
2. Pour the root beer into a large skillet, and heat it on high heat until it comes to a boil. Allow the coke to cook for about another 15 or 20 minutes, until the root beer reduces down to 1 cup of liquid. Let the liquid cool.
3. Place the milk and cream in a bowl, and mix them together until well combined. Use a whisk to mix in the sugar. Continue to whisk for about 4 minutes until the sugar dissolves. Then mix in the vanilla extract and root beer reduction and lemon juice.
4. Pour the ingredients into your ice cream maker, and let it churn for 25 minutes. About 5 minutes before the ice cream is done churning add the chocolate to your ice cream maker.
5. Put the gelato in an airtight container and place in the freezer for up to 2 hours, until desired consistency is reached.

Cookies 'n Cream Rice Crispy Treat Frozen Yogurt

Servings: 1 Quart
Cooking Time: 2 Hours 35 Minutes
Ingredients:
- 1 quart container full-fat plain yogurt
- ¼ teaspoon salt
- 1 cup sugar

- 1 teaspoon vanilla extract
- 10 chocolate sandwich cookies
- 1/2 cup rice crispy treats

Directions:
1. Refer to note at the beginning of the chapter about freezing bowl.
2. Place the yogurt in a bowl. Use a whisk to mix in the sugar and salt. Continue to whisk for about 4 minutes until the sugar dissolves. Then mix in the vanilla extract.
3. Place the sandwich cookies in a food processor, and process until the cookies are no bigger than chocolate chips. If you don't have a food processor place the cookies in a large resealable plastic bag, and seal it shut. Use your hands, a mallet, or a rolling pin to crush the cookies.
4. Pour the ingredients into your ice cream maker, and let it churn for 25 minutes. About 5 minutes before the ice cream is done churning add the cookies, and small chunks of the rice crispy treats to your ice cream maker.
5. Put the frozen yogurt in an airtight container and place in the freezer for at least 2 hours, until desired consistency is reached.

Double Espresso Ice Cream

Servings: 10
Cooking Time: 30 Minutes
Ingredients:
- 2 cups half and half
- 1 ½ cups heavy cream
- 14 ounces sweetened condensed milk
- 2 tablespoons espresso powder
- 6 egg yolks
- ¼ cup chocolate-covered espresso beans, chopped

Directions:
1. Add the half and half, cream, condensed milk, and espresso powder in a saucepan and heat over medium low flame. Simmer for 3 minutes. Remove from the stove.
2. In a bowl, whisk in the egg yolks. Drizzle ½ cup of the warm milk into the egg yolks while whisking constantly to form a smooth mixture. Whisk the egg mixture back into the pot.

3. Turn on the heat to medium low and cook until the mixture starts to thicken. Constantly stir while cooking.

4. Turn off the heat and strain the mixture to remove lumps. Allow to cool at room temperature. Place in the fridge to chill for 2 hours.

5. Turn on the Hamilton Beach and pour the mixture in. Churn for 15 minutes.

6. Five minutes before the time ends, add the chocolate-covered espresso beans.

7. Transfer to an airtight container.

8. Place in the fridge to completely cool.

Nutrition Info: Calories per serving:166 ; Protein: 4.8g; Carbs: 9.2g; Fat: 12.4g Sugar: 5.6g

Chocolate Cookie Rice Crispy Treat Frozen Yogurt

Servings: 1 Quart
Cooking Time: 2 Hours 35 Minutes
Ingredients:

- 1 quart container full-fat plain yogurt
- ¼ teaspoon salt
- 1 cup sugar
- 1 teaspoon vanilla extract
- 10 chocolate sandwich cookies
- 1/2 cup rice crispy treats
- ¼ cup milk chocolate (chopped fine)

Directions:

1. NOTE: Freeze your ice cream bowl for at least 24hrs prior to starting!

2. Place the yogurt in a bowl. Use a whisk to mix in the sugar and salt. Continue to whisk for about 4 minutes until the sugar dissolves. Then mix in the vanilla extract.

3. Place the sandwich cookies in a food processor, and process until the cookies are no bigger than chocolate chips. If you don't have a food processor place the cookies in a large resealable plastic bag, and seal it shut. Use your hands, a mallet, or a rolling pin to crush the cookies.

4. Pour the ingredients into your ice cream maker, and let it churn for 25 minutes. About 5 minutes before the ice cream is done churning add the cookies, and small chunks of the rice crispy treats to your ice cream maker.

5. Put the frozen yogurt in an airtight container and place in the freezer for at least 2 hours, until desired consistency is reached.

Butter Pecan Ice Cream

Servings: 10
Cooking Time: 25 Minutes
Ingredients:

- ½ cup unsalted butter
- 1 cup chopped pecan
- 1 teaspoon salt
- 1 cup ice cold whole milk
- ¾ cup granulated sugar
- 2 cups ice cold heavy cream
- 1 teaspoon pure vanilla extract

Directions:

1. Melt the butter in skillet and add the nuts and salt. Sauté over medium heat until the nuts are golden. Remove and strain the nuts. Reserve the butter for another use. Set aside the nuts. Allow the nuts to cool at least to room temperature.

2. Put ice water in a large mixing bowl. Place a small bowl on top of the large bowl with ice. Whisk in the milk and sugar until the sugar dissolves. Add the heavy cream and vanilla. Stir until combined.

3. Turn on the Hamilton Beach and pour the mixture in. Freeze for 25 minutes and add the nuts five minutes before the time ends.

4. Place the ice cream into a container and freeze overnight.

Nutrition Info: Calories per serving: 281; Protein: 4.6g; Carbs:10.2 g; Fat: 25.4g Sugar: 9g

THE CLASSICS ICE CREAM

Kahlua & Pistachio Ice Cream

Servings: 6
Cooking Time: 2 Hours 50 Minutes
Ingredients:
- 2 cups heavy cream
- 1 cup milk
- 3/4 cup sugar
- 1 teaspoon vanilla extract
- 3 tablespoons Kahlua
- 3/4 cup chops almond

Directions:
1. NOTE: Freeze your ice cream bowl for at least 24hrs prior to starting!
2. Place the milk and cream in a bowl, and mix them together until well combined. Use a whisk to mix in the sugar. Continue to whisk for about 4 minutes until the sugar dissolves. Then mix in the vanilla extract, Kahlua.
3. Pour the ingredients into your ice cream maker, and let it churn for 25 minutes. About 5 minutes before the ice cream is done churning add the almonds to your ice cream maker.
4. Put the ice cream in an airtight container and place in the freezer for around 2 hours. Allow the ice cream to thaw for 15 minutes before serving.

Double Gin And Tonic Soft Serve Ice Cream

Servings: 6
Cooking Time: 35 Minutes
Ingredients:
- 2 cups heavy cream
- 1 cup milk
- 3/4 cup sugar
- 1 Tbs. vanilla extract
- 4 tablespoons gin
- 125 ML tonic water

Directions:
1. Refer to note at the beginning of the chapter about freezing bowl.
2. Place the milk and cream in a bowl, and mix them together until well combined. Use a whisk to mix in the sugar. Continue to whisk for about 4 minutes until the sugar dissolves. Mix in the vanilla extract. Then whisk in the gin and tonic
3. Pour the ingredients into your ice cream maker, and let it churn for 25 minutes.
4. Serve immediately.

Miraculous Double Mint Chip Ice Cream

Servings: 6
Cooking Time: 2 Hours 50 Minutes
Ingredients:
- 2 cups heavy cream
- 1 cup milk
- 3/4 cup sugar
- 1 teaspoon vanilla extract
- 1 teaspoon peppermint extract
- 1 cup semi-sweet chocolate chips

Directions:
1. Refer to note at the beginning of the chapter about freezing bowl.
2. Place the milk and cream in a bowl, and mix them together until well combined. Use a whisk to mix in the sugar. Continue to whisk for about 4 minutes until the sugar dissolves. Then mix in the vanilla and peppermint extract.
3. Pour the ingredients into your ice cream maker, and let it churn for 25 minutes. About 5 minutes before the ice cream is finished churning, add in the chocolate chips.
4. Put the ice cream in an airtight container and place in the freezer for around 2 hours. Allow the ice cream to thaw for 15 minutes before serving.

"adults Old Fashioned" Ice Cream

Servings: 6
Cooking Time: 2 Hours 50 Minutes
Ingredients:
- 2 cups heavy cream
- 1 cup milk
- 3/4 cup sugar
- 1 tablespoon vanilla extract
- 3 tablespoons whiskey
- 1 dash of bitters

Directions:

1. Refer to note at the beginning of the chapter about freezing bowl.

2. Place the milk and cream in a bowl, and mix them together until well combined. Use a whisk to mix in the sugar. Continue to whisk for about 4 minutes until the sugar dissolves. Then mix in the vanilla extract, whiskey, and bitters.

3. Pour the ingredients into your ice cream maker, and let it churn for 25 minutes.

4. Put the ice cream in an airtight container and place in the freezer for around 2 hours. Allow the ice cream to thaw for 15 minutes before serving.

Chocolate Screwdriver Soft Serve Ice Cream

Servings: 6
Cooking Time: 35 Minutes
Ingredients:

- 2 cups heavy cream
- 1 cup milk
- 3/4 cup sugar
- 1 Tbs. vanilla extract
- 1 tbsp. coco powder
- ½ cup orange juice
- 3 tablespoons vodka

Directions:

1. NOTE: Freeze your ice cream bowl for at least 24hrs prior to starting!

2. Place the milk and cream in a bowl, and mix them together until well combined. Use a whisk to mix in the sugar. Continue to whisk for about 4 minutes until the sugar dissolves. Mix in the vanilla extract and coco powder. Then mix in the orange juice. Finally whisk in the vodka.

3. Pour the ingredients into your ice cream maker, and let it churn for 25 minutes.

4. Serve immediately.

The Guinness Chocolate Milkshake

Servings: 6
Cooking Time: 25 Minutes
Ingredients:

- 2 cups heavy cream
- 1 cup milk
- 3/4 cup sugar
- 3 tablespoons Guinness beer
- 4 ounces chopped semi-sweet chocolate

Directions:

1. Refer to note at the beginning of the chapter about freezing bowl.

2. Melt the chocolate, and let it cool for a bit.

3. Place the milk and cream in a bowl, and mix them together until well combined. Use a whisk to mix in the sugar. Continue to whisk for about 4 minutes until the sugar dissolves. Then mix in the chocolate and Guinness.

4. Pour the ingredients into your ice cream maker, and let it churn for 10-15 minutes, until desired consistency is reached. About 5 minutes before the ice cream is done churning add the peanut butter cup to your ice cream maker.

5. Serve immediately.

Chunky Chocolate Chip Soft Serve Ice Cream

Servings: 6
Cooking Time: 35 Minutes
Ingredients:

- 2 cups heavy cream
- 1 cup milk
- 3/4 cup sugar
- 1 Tbs. vanilla extract
- 1 cup chocolate chips of your choice

Directions:

1. Refer to note at the beginning of the chapter about freezing bowl.

2. Place the milk and cream in a bowl, and mix them together until well combined. Use a whisk to mix in the sugar. Continue to whisk for about 4 minutes until the sugar dissolves. Then mix in the vanilla extract.

3. Pour the ingredients into your ice cream maker, and let it churn for 25 minutes. About 5 minutes before the ice cream is finished churning, add in the chocolate chips.

4. Serve immediately.

Mint Cookies 'n Cream "silkshake"

Servings: 6
Cooking Time: 25 Minutes
Ingredients:

- 2 cups heavy cream
- 1 cup milk
- 3/4 cup sugar
- 1 teaspoon vanilla extract
- 1 ½ teaspoons mint extract
- 10 chocolate sandwich cookies

Directions:
1.   Refer to note at the beginning of the chapter about freezing bowl.
2.   Place the milk and cream in a bowl, and mix them together until well combined. Use a whisk to mix in the sugar. Continue to whisk for about 4 minutes until the sugar dissolves. Then mix in the vanilla and mint extract.
3.   Place the sandwich cookies in a food processor, and process until the cookies are no bigger than chocolate chips. If you don't have a food processor place the cookies in a large resealable plastic bag, and seal it shut. Use your hands, a mallet, or a rolling pin to crush the cookies.
4.   Pour the ingredients into your ice cream maker, and let it churn for 10-15 minutes, until desired consistency is reached. About 5 minutes before the ice cream is done churning add the cookies to your ice cream maker.
5.   Serve immediately.

Radical Rocky Road Ice Cream

Servings: 6
Cooking Time: 2 Hours 50 Minutes
Ingredients:

- 2 cups heavy cream
- 1 cup milk
- 3/4 cup sugar
- 1 Tbs. vanilla extract
- ½ cup unsweetened cocoa powder
- ½ cup chopped pecans
- 1 cup mini marshmallows

Directions:
1.   Refer to note at the beginning of the chapter about freezing bowl.
2.   Place the milk and cream in a bowl, and mix them together until well combined. Use a whisk to mix in the sugar. Continue to whisk for about 4 minutes until the sugar dissolves. Then whisk in cocoa powder until all lumps are gone, and well mixed. Then mix in the vanilla extract.
3.   Pour the ingredients into your ice cream maker, and let it churn for 25 minutes. About 5 minutes before the ice cream is finished churning, add in the pecans and marshmallows.
4.   Put the ice cream in an airtight container and place in the freezer for around 2 hours. Allow the ice cream to thaw for 15 minutes before serving.

The Original "manhattan" Ice Cream

Servings: 6
Cooking Time: 2 Hours 50 Minutes
Ingredients:

- 2 cups heavy cream
- 1 cup milk
- 3/4 cup sugar
- 1 tablespoon vanilla extract
- 3 tablespoons whiskey
- 1 tablespoon vermouth
- 1 dash of bitters

Directions:
1.   NOTE: Freeze your ice cream bowl for at least 24hrs prior to starting!
2.   Place the milk and cream in a bowl, and mix them together until well combined. Use a whisk to mix in the sugar. Continue to whisk for about 4 minutes until the sugar dissolves. Then mix in the vanilla extract, whiskey, vermouth, and bitters.
3.   Pour the ingredients into your ice cream maker, and let it churn for 25 minutes.
4.   Put the ice cream in an airtight container and place in the freezer for around 2 hours. Allow the ice cream to thaw for 15 minutes before serving.

Creamy Kahlua Almond Delight Ice Cream

Servings: 6
Cooking Time: 2 Hours 50 Minutes
Ingredients:

- 2 cups heavy cream

- 1 cup milk
- 3/4 cup sugar
- 1 teaspoon vanilla extract
- 3 tablespoons kahlua
- 3/4 cup chops almond

Directions:

1. Refer to note at the beginning of the chapter about freezing bowl.
2. Place the milk and cream in a bowl, and mix them together until well combined. Use a whisk to mix in the sugar. Continue to whisk for about 4 minutes until the sugar dissolves. Then mix in the vanilla extract, kahlua.
3. Pour the ingredients into your ice cream maker, and let it churn for 25 minutes. About 5 minutes before the ice cream is done churning add the almonds to your ice cream maker.
4. Put the ice cream in an airtight container and place in the freezer for around 2 hours. Allow the ice cream to thaw for 15 minutes before serving.

Sunrise Strawberry Daiquiri Milkshake

Servings: 6
Cooking Time: 25 Minutes
Ingredients:

- 2 cups heavy cream
- 1 cup milk
- 3/4 cup sugar
- 4 tablespoons rum
- 8 ounces strawberries

Directions:

1. Refer to note at the beginning of the chapter about freezing bowl.
2. Puree the strawberries in a food processor or blender.
3. Place the milk and cream in a bowl, and mix them together until well combined. Use a whisk to mix in the sugar. Continue to whisk for about 4 minutes until the sugar dissolves. Then mix in the rum, and strawberry puree.
4. Pour the ingredients into your ice cream maker, and let it churn for 10-15 minutes, until desired consistency is reached. About 5 minutes before the ice cream is done churning add the peanut butter cup to your ice cream maker.

5. Serve immediately.

Power Punch Pistachio Ice Cream

Servings: 6
Cooking Time: 2 Hours 50 Minutes
Ingredients:

- 2 cups heavy cream
- 1 cup milk
- 3/4 cup sugar
- 1/4 teaspoon almond extract
- 1/2 cup chopped pistachios

Directions:

1. Refer to note at the beginning of the chapter about freezing bowl.
2. Place the milk and cream in a bowl, and mix them together until well combined. Use a whisk to mix in the sugar. Continue to whisk for about 4 minutes until the sugar dissolves. Then mix in the almond extract.
3. Pour the ingredients into your ice cream maker, and let it churn for 25 minutes. About 5 minutes before the ice cream is finished churning, add in the pistachios.
4. Put the ice cream in an airtight container and place in the freezer for around 2 hours. Allow the ice cream to thaw for 15 minutes before serving.

"the Big Stout" Almond Chocolate Milkshake

Servings: 6
Cooking Time: 25 Minutes
Ingredients:

- 2 cups heavy cream
- 1 cup milk
- 3/4 cup sugar
- 4 ounces chopped semi-sweet chocolate
- 3 tablespoons almonds
- 3 tablespoons Guinness beer

Directions:

1. NOTE: Freeze your ice cream bowl for at least 24hrs prior to starting!
2. Melt the chocolate, and let it cool for a bit.
3. Place the milk and cream in a bowl, and mix them together until well combined. Use a whisk to

mix in the sugar. Continue to whisk for about 4 minutes until the sugar dissolves. Then mix in the chocolate and Guinness.

4. Pour the ingredients into your ice cream maker, and let it churn for 10-15 minutes, until desired consistency is reached. About 5 minutes before the ice cream is done churning add the almonds to your ice cream maker.

5. Serve immediately.

Classic Vanilla Soft-serve Ice Cream

Servings: 6
Cooking Time: 35 Minutes
Ingredients:
- 2 cups heavy cream
- 1 cup milk
- 3/4 cup sugar
- 1 Tbs. vanilla extract

Directions:
1. Refer to note at the beginning of the chapter about freezing bowl.
2. Place the milk and cream in a bowl, and mix them together until well combined. Use a whisk to mix in the sugar. Continue to whisk for about 4 minutes until the sugar dissolves. Then mix in the vanilla extract.
3. Pour the ingredients into your ice cream maker, and let it churn for 25 minutes.
4. Serve immediately.

Grown Folks "old Fashioned" Ice Cream

Servings: 6
Cooking Time: 2 Hours 50 Minutes
Ingredients:
- 2 cups heavy cream
- 1 cup milk
- 3/4 cup sugar
- 1 tablespoon vanilla extract
- 3 tablespoons whiskey
- 1 dash of bitters

Directions:

1. NOTE: Freeze your ice cream bowl for at least 24hrs prior to starting!
2. Place the milk and cream in a bowl, and mix them together until well combined. Use a whisk to mix in the sugar. Continue to whisk for about 4 minutes until the sugar dissolves. Then mix in the vanilla extract, whiskey, and bitters.
3. Pour the ingredients into your ice cream maker, and let it churn for 25 minutes.
4. Put the ice cream in an airtight container and place in the freezer for around 2 hours. Allow the ice cream to thaw for 15 minutes before serving.

Pralines And "oh So Creamy" Milkshake

Servings: 6
Cooking Time: 25 Minutes
Ingredients:
- 2 cups heavy cream
- 1 cup milk
- 1 cup brown sugar
- 1 teaspoon vanilla extract
- 1/3 cup finely chopped pecans
- 1 tablespoon butter

Directions:
1. Refer to note at the beginning of the chapter about freezing bowl.
2. Melt the butter in a small skillet on medium heat. Add the pecans, and cook for about 5 minutes, until they become lightly browned.
3. Place the milk and cream in a bowl, and mix them together until well combined. Use a whisk to mix in the sugar. Continue to whisk for about 4 minutes until the sugar dissolves. Then mix in the vanilla extract.
4. Pour the ingredients into your ice cream maker, and let it churn for 10-15 minutes, until desired consistency is reached. About 5 minutes before the ice cream is done churning add the cookie dough to your ice cream maker.
5. Serve immediately.

Tropical Coconut Rum And Coke Gelato

Servings: 4-6
Cooking Time: 2 Hours 50 Minutes
Ingredients:

- 1/2 cup heavy cream
- 2 cups milk
- 3/4 cup sugar
- 1 teaspoon vanilla extract
- 3 tablespoons rum
- ¼ cup shaved coconut
- 3 cups coca cola (2, 12 ounce cans)

Directions:

1. NOTE: Freeze your ice cream bowl for at least 24hrs prior to starting!
2. Pour the coke into a large skillet, and heat it on high heat until it comes to a boil. Allow the coke to cook for about another 15 or 20 minutes, until the coke reduces down to 1 cup of liquid. Let the liquid cool.
3. Place the milk and cream in a bowl, and mix them together until well combined. Use a whisk to mix in the sugar. Continue to whisk for about 4 minutes until the sugar dissolves. Then mix in the vanilla extract, coke reduction, coconut chips and rum.
4. Pour the ingredients into your ice cream maker, and let it churn for 25 minutes.
5. Put the gelato in an airtight container and place in the freezer for up to 2 hours, until desired consistency is reached.

Daiquiri Lime Soda Frozen Yogurt

Servings: 1 Quart
Cooking Time: 2 Hours 35 Minutes
Ingredients:

- 1 quart container full-fat plain yogurt
- ¼ teaspoon salt
- 1 cup sugar
- 1/4 cup lime juice
- ¼ cup sprite
- 4 tablespoons rum

Directions:

1. NOTE: Freeze your ice cream bowl for at least 24hrs prior to starting!
2. Place the yogurt in a bowl. Use a whisk to mix in the sugar and salt. Continue to whisk for about 4 minutes until the sugar dissolves. Then mix in the rum, and lime juice.
3. Pour the ingredients into your ice cream maker, and let it churn for 25 minutes.
4. Put the frozen yogurt in an airtight container and place in the freezer for at least 2 hours, until desired consistency is reached.

Caribbean Colada Frozen Yogurt

Servings: 1 Quart
Cooking Time: 2 Hours 35 Minutes
Ingredients:

- 1 quart container full-fat plain yogurt
- ¼ teaspoon salt
- 1 cup sugar
- ½ cup pineapple juice
- 1 drop coconut essence
- 2 teaspoons lime juice
- 1/4 cup shredded coconut
- 4 tablespoons rum

Directions:

1. NOTE: Freeze your ice cream bowl for at least 24hrs prior to starting!
2. Place the yogurt in a bowl. Use a whisk to mix in the sugar and salt. Continue to whisk for about 4 minutes until the sugar dissolves. Then mix in the rum, pineapple juice, lime juice, and coconut essence.
3. Pour the ingredients into your ice cream maker, and let it churn for 25 minutes. About 5 minutes before the ice cream is done churning add the shredded coconut to your ice cream maker.
4. Put the frozen yogurt in an airtight container and place in the freezer for at least 2 hours, until desired consistency is reached.

Tropical Watermelon Lemon/lime Sorbet

Servings: Makes 1 Quart
Cooking Time: 2 Hours 40 Minutes

Ingredients:

- 3 1/2 cups sliced seedless watermelon
- 6-ounce chilled pineapple juice
- 3/4 cup chilled ginger ale
- ½ cup fresh lime juice
- 1/3 cup grenadine

Directions:

1. NOTE: Freeze your ice cream bowl for at least 24hrs prior to starting!
2. Puree all ingredients in a food processor or blender.
3. Pour the ingredients into your ice cream maker, and let it churn for 25-30 minutes.
4. Place in an airtight container for up to 2 hours, until desired consistency is reached.

Lickin' Lime Daiquiri Frozen Yogurt

Servings: 1 Quart
Cooking Time: 2 Hours 35 Minutes

Ingredients:

- 1 quart container full-fat plain yogurt
- ¼ teaspoon salt
- 1 cup sugar
- 1/3 cup lime juice
- 4 tablespoons rum

Directions:

1. Refer to note at the beginning of the chapter about freezing bowl.
2. Place the yogurt in a bowl. Use a whisk to mix in the sugar and salt. Continue to whisk for about 4 minutes until the sugar dissolves. Then mix in the rum, and lime juice.
3. Pour the ingredients into your ice cream maker, and let it churn for 25 minutes.
4. Put the frozen yogurt in an airtight container and place in the freezer for at least 2 hours, until desired consistency is reached.

Chocolate Chip Cookie Dough Frozen Yogurt

Servings: 1 Quart
Cooking Time: 2 Hours 35 Minutes

Ingredients:

- 1 quart container full-fat plain yogurt
- ¼ teaspoon salt
- 1 cup sugar
- 1 tablespoon vanilla extract
- ½ cup prepackaged cookie dough cut into small chunks

Directions:

1. Refer to note at the beginning of the chapter about freezing bowl.
2. Place the yogurt in a bowl. Use a whisk to mix in the sugar and salt. Continue to whisk for about 4 minutes until the sugar dissolves. Then mix in the vanilla extract.
3. Pour the ingredients into your ice cream maker, and let it churn for 25 minutes. About 5 minutes before the ice cream is done churning add the cookie dough to your ice cream maker.
4. Put the frozen yogurt in an airtight container and place in the freezer for at least 2 hours, until desired consistency is reached.

Double Dark Chocolate Gelato

Servings: 4-6
Cooking Time: 2 Hours 35 Minutes

Ingredients:

- 12 cup heavy cream
- 2 cups milk
- 34 cup sugar
- 14 teaspoon salt
- 7 ounces high quality dark chocolate
- 1 teaspoon vanilla extract

Directions:

1. Refer to note at the beginning of the chapter about freezing bowl.
2. Melt the chocolate, and allow it to cool a little bit.
3. Place the milk and cream in a bowl, and mix them together until well combined. Use a whisk to mix in the sugar and salt. Continue to whisk for about 4 minutes until the sugar and salt dissolve. Then mix in the vanilla extract. Finally mix in the chocolate until well combined.

4. Pour the ingredients into your ice cream maker, and let it churn for 25 minutes.

5. Put the gelato in an airtight container and place in the freezer for up to 2 hours, until desired consistency is reached.

Orange Tequila "sunrise" Gelato

Servings: 4-6
Cooking Time: 2 Hours 35 Minutes
Ingredients:
- 1/2 cup heavy cream
- 2 cups milk
- 3/4 cup sugar
- I/2 cup orange juice
- 1 teaspoon vanilla extract
- 3 tablespoons tequila
- ½ tablespoon grenadine

Directions:
1. NOTE: Freeze your ice cream bowl for at least 24hrs prior to starting!
2. Place the milk and cream in a bowl, and mix them together until well combined. Use a whisk to mix in the sugar. Continue to whisk for about 4 minutes until the sugar dissolves. Then mix in the vanilla extract, orange juice, tequila and grenadine.
3. Pour the ingredients into your ice cream maker, and let it churn for 25 minutes.
4. Put the gelato in an airtight container and place in the freezer for up to 2 hours, until desired consistency is reached.

Margarita Madness Soft Serve Ice Cream

Servings: 6
Cooking Time: 35 Minutes
Ingredients:
- 2 cups heavy cream
- 1 cup milk
- 3/4 cup sugar
- 1 Tbs. vanilla extract
- 3 tablespoons tequila
- 1/2 cup lime juice
- 2 tablespoons orange liqueur

Directions:
1. Refer to note at the beginning of the chapter about freezing bowl.
2. Place the milk and cream in a bowl, and mix them together until well combined. Use a whisk to mix in the sugar. Continue to whisk for about 4 minutes until the sugar dissolves. Mix in the vanilla extract. Finally whisk in the lime juice, tequila, and liqueur.
3. Pour the ingredients into your ice cream maker, and let it churn for 25 minutes.
4. Serve immediately.

"new York" Manhattan Ice Cream

Servings: 6
Cooking Time: 2 Hours 50 Minutes
Ingredients:
- 2 cups heavy cream
- 1 cup milk
- 3/4 cup sugar
- 1 tablespoon vanilla extract
- 3 tablespoons whiskey
- 1 tablespoon vermouth
- 1 dash of bitters

Directions:
1. Refer to note at the beginning of the chapter about freezing bowl.
2. Place the milk and cream in a bowl, and mix them together until well combined. Use a whisk to mix in the sugar. Continue to whisk for about 4 minutes until the sugar dissolves. Then mix in the vanilla extract, whiskey, vermouth, and bitters.
3. Pour the ingredients into your ice cream maker, and let it churn for 25 minutes.
4. Put the ice cream in an airtight container and place in the freezer for around 2 hours. Allow the ice cream to thaw for 15 minutes before serving.

Strawberry Cinnamon Margarita Soft Serve Ice Cream

Servings: 6
Cooking Time: 35 Minutes

Ingredients:

- 2 cups heavy cream
- 1 cup milk
- 3/4 cup sugar
- 1 Tbs. vanilla extract
- 3 tablespoons tequila
- 1 tablespoon cinnamon
- 1/2 cup lime juice
- ¼ cup strawberries (mashed up)
- 2 tablespoons orange liqueur

Directions:

1. NOTE: Freeze your ice cream bowl for at least 24hrs prior to starting!
2. Place the milk and cream in a bowl, and mix them together until well combined. Use a whisk to mix in the sugar and cinnamon. Continue to whisk for about 4 minutes until the sugar dissolves. Mix the vanilla extract and whisk in the lime juice, strawberries, tequila, and liqueur.
3. Pour the ingredients into your ice cream maker, and let it churn for 25 minutes.
4. Serve immediately.

OTHER FAVORITE RECIPES

Pumpkin Cinnamon Raisin Gingerbread Frozen Yogurt

Servings: 1 Quart
Cooking Time: 2 Hours 35 Minutes
Ingredients:

- 1 quart container full-fat plain yogurt
- ¼ teaspoon salt
- 1 cup sugar
- 1 teaspoon vanilla extract
- 1/2 cup pumpkin
- ¼ cup raisins
- 2 tablespoons molasses
- 1 teaspoon cinnamon
- ¼ teaspoon ginger

Directions:

1. NOTE: Freeze your ice cream bowl for at least 24hrs prior to starting!
2. Place all the ingredients in a blender and blend on high until pureed and sugar dissolves.
3. Pour the ingredients into your ice cream maker, and let it churn for 25 minutes. About 5 minutes before the ice cream is done churning add the raisins to your ice cream maker.
4. Put the frozen yogurt in an airtight container and place in the freezer for at least 2 hours, until desired consistency is reached.

Banana Pineapple Coconut Gelato

Servings: 4-6
Cooking Time: 2 Hours 35 Minutes
Ingredients:

- 1/2 cup heavy cream
- 2 cups milk
- 3/4 cup sugar
- 1 tablespoon vanilla extract
- ½ cup sliced banana
- ½ cup chopped pineapple
- ½ cup chopped coconut

Directions:

1. NOTE: Freeze your ice cream bowl for at least 24hrs prior to starting!
2. Puree the bananas in a food processor or blender.
3. Place the milk and cream in a bowl, and mix them together until well combined. Use a whisk to mix in the sugar. Continue to whisk for about 4 minutes until the sugar dissolves. Then mix in the vanilla extract and banana puree.
4. Pour the ingredients into your ice cream maker, and let it churn for 25 minutes. About 5 minutes before the ice cream is done churning add the walnuts to your ice cream maker.
5. Put the gelato in an airtight container and place in the freezer for up to 2 hours, until desired consistency is reached.

Amazing Key Lime Sorbet

Servings: 4
Cooking Time: 3 Hours
Ingredients:

- 3 cups cold water
- 2 ¼ cup fresh key lime juice
- 2 3/4 cup sugar
- 1 tablespoon lime zest

Directions:

1. NOTE: Freeze your ice cream bowl for at least 24hrs prior to starting!
2. Mix together the water and sugar in a large sauce pan on medium heat. Allow the mixture to come to a boil. Then lower to low heat, and let the mixture simmer until the sugar dissolve. Allow the mixture to cool completely.
3. Mix the lime juice and zest with the cooled mixture.
4. Pour the ingredients into your ice cream maker, and let it churn for 25-30 minutes.
5. Place in an airtight container for up to 2 hours, until desired consistency is reached.

Peach Sorbet

Servings: 8
Cooking Time: 15 Minutes
Ingredients:

- 2/3 cup sugar
- 1 cup water

- 2 ½ pounds peaches, peeled and halved (seeds removed)
- 3 tablespoons fresh lemon juice
- ½ teaspoon lemon zest

Directions:
1. Place sugar and water in a saucepan. Bring to a boil until the sugar dissolves. Add the peaches and simmer for another 3 minutes.
2. Remove from the heat and place in the fridge to chill for at least 3 hours.
3. Place all ingredients in a blender and add the chilled sugar mixture. Pulse until smooth. Allow to chill for another two hours.
4. Turn on the Hamilton Beach and pour in the mixture.
5. Churn for 10 minutes.
6. Transfer in an airtight container and freeze overnight.

Nutrition Info: Calories per serving: 121; Protein: 1g; Carbs: 31g; Fat: 0g Sugar: 25g

Frozen Cantaloupe Yogurt

Servings: 6
Cooking Time: 10 Minutes
Ingredients:
- 3 cups non-fat Greek yogurt
- 2/3 cup white sugar
- 1teaspoon vanilla extract
- 1 cup cantaloupe flesh

Directions:
1. Place all ingredients in a food processor. Pulse until smooth.
2. Turn on the Hamilton Beach and pour in the mixture.
3. Churn for 10 minutes.
4. Transfer in an airtight container and freeze overnight.

Nutrition Info: Calories per serving: 126; Protein: 9.3g; Carbs: 21.7g; Fat: 0.3g Sugar: 20g

Matcha Frozen Yogurt

Servings: 6
Cooking Time: 10 Minutes
Ingredients:

- 2 cups Greek yogurt
- ¾ cup sugar
- 2 tablespoons matcha powder
- A pinch of salt

Directions:
1. In a cold bowl, combine all ingredients.
2. Turn on the Hamilton Beach and pour in the mixture.
3. Churn for 10 minutes.
4. Transfer in an airtight container and freeze overnight.

Nutrition Info: Calories per serving: 106; Protein: 3.1g; Carbs: 18.1g; Fat: 2.7g Sugar: 16.2g

Cherry Chocolate Pretzel Gelato

Servings: 4-6
Cooking Time: 2 Hours 35 Minutes
Ingredients:
- 1/2 cup heavy cream
- 2 cups milk
- 3/4 cup sugar
- 1 teaspoon vanilla extract
- 2 ounces pitted cherries
- 3 ounces semi-sweet chocolate
- 4 ounce pretzels

Directions:
1. NOTE: Freeze your ice cream bowl for at least 24hrs prior to starting!
2. Melt the chocolate, and allow it to cool a little bit.
3. Place the milk and cream in a bowl, and mix them together until well combined. Use a whisk to mix in the sugar. Continue to whisk for about 4 minutes until the sugar dissolves. Then mix in the vanilla extract. Finally mix in the chocolate and cherries.
4. Place the pretzels in a food processor, and process until the cookies are no bigger than chocolate chips. If you don't have a food processor place the pretzels in a large resealable plastic bag, and seal it shut. Use your hands, a mallet, or a rolling pin to crush the pretzels.
5. Pour the ingredients into your ice cream maker, and let it churn for 25 minutes. About 5 minutes before the ice cream is done churning add the pretzels to your ice cream maker.

6. Put the gelato in an airtight container and place in the freezer for up to 2 hours, until desired consistency is reached.

Watermelon Sorbet

Servings: 7
Cooking Time: 15 Minutes
Ingredients:
- 1 cup sugar
- 1 cup water
- ¼ cup lemon juice
- 3 cups watermelon, peeled and seeded

Directions:
1. Place the water and sugar in a saucepan and bring to a boil over medium heat until the sugar dissolves. Remove from the heat and place in the fridge to chill for at least 3 hours.
2. Once cooled, place the water-sugar mixture into a blender and add the rest of the ingredients. Pulse until smooth.
3. Turn on the Hamilton Beach and pour in the mixture.
4. Churn for 10 minutes.
5. Transfer in an airtight container and freeze overnight.

Nutrition Info: Calories per serving: 77; Protein: 0.4g; Carbs: 19.8g; Fat: 0.1g Sugar: 12.3g

"crispy" Kit Kat Ice Cream

Servings: 6
Cooking Time: 2 Hours 50 Minutes
Ingredients:
- 2 cups heavy cream
- 1 cup milk
- 3/4 cup sugar
- 1 tablespoon vanilla extract
- 1 ½ cups chopped mini kit kats

Directions:
1. Refer to note at the beginning of the chapter about freezing bowl.
2. Place the milk and cream in a bowl, and mix them together until well combined. Use a whisk to mix in the sugar. Continue to whisk for about 4

minutes until the sugar dissolves. Then mix in the vanilla extract.
3. Pour the ingredients into your ice cream maker, and let it churn for 25 minutes. About 5 minutes before the ice cream is done churning add the kit kats to your ice cream maker.
4. Put the ice cream in an airtight container and place in the freezer for around 2 hours. Allow the ice cream to thaw for 15 minutes before serving.

Grape Sorbet

Servings: 6
Cooking Time: 10 Minutes
Ingredients:
- 4 cups seedless grapes
- 1/3 cup granulated sugar
- 2 tablespoon lemon juice

Directions:
1. Place the grapes and sugar in a blender and pulse until smooth.
2. Pass the mixture through a sieve to remove the skin.
3. Add the lemon juice to the grape puree.
4. Turn on the Hamilton Beach and pour in the mixture.
5. Churn for 10 minutes.
6. Transfer in an airtight container and freeze overnight.

Nutrition Info: Calories per serving: 100; Protein: 1g; Carbs: 26g; Fat: 0g Sugar: 18g

Neapolitan Frozen Yogurt

Servings: 10
Cooking Time: 10 Minutes
Ingredients:
- 1 cup cherries, pitted
- ½ cup icing sugar
- 1 lemon, juiced
- 2 cups plain Greek yogurt
- ½ cup frozen mango chunks
- 2 tablespoons honey
- ¼ cup frozen blueberries
- Mint leaves for garnish

Directions:

1. Place the cherries, icing sugar, and lemon juice in a food processor. Pulse until smooth.
2. Place in a bowl and add the yogurt. Allow to chill in the fridge for 30 minutes.
3. Turn on the Hamilton Beach and pour in the mixture.
4. Churn for 10 minutes.
5. Five minutes before churning ends, add the mango, honey, and blueberries.
6. Transfer in an airtight container and freeze overnight.
7. Serve with mint.

Nutrition Info: Calories per serving: 66; Protein: 2.1g; Carbs: 10.9g; Fat: 2g Sugar: 9.4g

Raspberry Lavender Sorbet

Servings: 6
Cooking Time: 5 Hours 35 Minutes
Ingredients:
- 3 cups, mashed raspberries
- ½ teaspoon lavender
- 3/4 cup sugar
- 1/2 teaspoon salt
- 2 tablespoons vanilla extract
- 2 ½ teaspoons lime juice

Directions:
1. NOTE: Freeze your ice cream bowl for at least 24hrs prior to starting!
2. Use a food processor or blender to puree the lavender, sugar, raspberries, and vanilla extract. Then blend in the salt and lime juice. Strain the mixture into a bowl, and refrigerate covered for 2-3 hours.
3. Pour the ingredients into your ice cream maker, and let it churn for 25-30 minutes.
4. Place in an airtight container for up to 2 hours, until desired consistency is reached.

Vegan Chunky Chocolate Banana Milkshake

Servings: 9
Cooking Time: 40 Minutes
Ingredients:
- 3/4 cup water

- 1 1/4 cups full fat coconut milk or coconut cream (as thick as possible)
- 2/3 cup organic cane sugar
- 2/3 cup unsweetened cocoa powder
- 1/4 tsp sea salt
- 6 ounces vegan dark chocolate, finely chopped
- 1/2 tsp pure vanilla extract
- ½ cup sliced frozen bananas

Directions:
1. Refer to note at the beginning of the chapter about freezing bowl.
2. Put the first 5 ingredients in a large saucepan, and heat it on medium-high heat. Mix the ingredients together using a whisk. Allow the mixture to come to a low boil. Continue to whisk often, and remain cooking on a low boil for 1 minute.
3. Take the pan off the heat, and mix in the chocolate and vanilla extract using the whisk. Continue to mix until the chocolate is melted.
4. Place the mixture in a blender with the bananas, and blend on high speed for about 30 seconds.
5. Allow the mixture to cool
6. Pour the ingredients into your ice cream maker, and let it churn for 10-15 minutes, until desired consistency is reached.
7. Serve immediately.

Honey Peach Gelato

Servings: 4-6
Cooking Time: 2 Hours 35 Minutes
Ingredients:
- 1/2 cup heavy cream
- 2 cups milk
- 3/4 cup sugar
- 1 cup sliced peaches
- 1 tablespoon vanilla extract
- 1/4 cup honey

Directions:
1. NOTE: Freeze your ice cream bowl for at least 24hrs prior to starting!
2. Puree the peaches in a food processor or blender.
3. Place the milk and cream in a bowl, and mix them together until well combined. Use a whisk to mix in the sugar. Continue to whisk for about 4

minutes until the sugar dissolves. Then mix in the vanilla extract honey and peach puree.

4.   Pour the ingredients into your ice cream maker, and let it churn for 25 minutes.

5.   Put the gelato in an airtight container and place in the freezer for up to 2 hours, until desired consistency is reached.

Lemon Scented Rose Gelato

Servings: 4-6
Cooking Time: 2 Hours 35 Minutes
Ingredients:

- 1/2 cup heavy cream
- 2 cups milk
- 3/4 cup sugar
- 1 teaspoon rose extract
- juice of ½ lemon

Directions:

1.   NOTE: Freeze your ice cream bowl for at least 24hrs prior to starting!

2.   Place the milk and cream in a bowl, and mix them together until well combined. Use a whisk to mix in the sugar. Continue to whisk for about 4 minutes until the sugar dissolves. Then mix in the rose extract.

3.   Pour the ingredients into your ice cream maker, and let it churn for 25 minutes.

4.   Put the gelato in an airtight container and place in the freezer for up to 2 hours, until desired consistency is reached.

Wonderful Watermelon Sorbet

Servings: Makes 1 Quart
Cooking Time: 2 Hours 40 Minutes
Ingredients:

- 3 1/2 cups sliced seedless watermelon
- 6 ounce chilled pineapple juice
- 3/4 cup chilled ginger ale
- ½ cup fresh lime juice
- 1/3 cup grenadine

Directions:

1.   Refer to note at the beginning of the chapter about freezing bowl.

2.   Puree all ingredients in a food processor or blender.

3.   Pour the ingredients into your ice cream maker, and let it churn for 25-30 minutes.

4.   Place in an airtight container for up to 2 hours, until desired consistency is reached.

Succulent Waffle Cookie Ice Cream Sandwich

Servings: 6
Cooking Time: 5 Minutes
Ingredients:

- 1 cup flour
- 1 tbsp. sugar
- 2 tsp. baking powder
- ½ tsp. cinnamon
- ¼ tsp. salt
- 1 egg
- 1 cup milk
- 1 ½ tbs. melted butter

Directions:

1.   Crack eggs and mix in a bowl with salt and pepper.

2.   Pour 2 tbsps. Milk to the eggs and whisk. Mix in the other ingredients until the batter is smooth.

3.   Spray your waffle maker with oil. Pour 2 tbsp. batter into the waffle maker and cook until crispy. Repeat until all the batter is used.

4.   Put a scoop of ice cream (that you made from this book) in the middle of two waffles.

5.   Drizzle honey over the top for a sweeter experience.

Watermelon Strawberry Frozen Yogurt

Servings: 12
Cooking Time: 10 Minutes
Ingredients:

- 1 cup watermelon, cubed and seeds removed
- 2 cups frozen strawberries, hulled
- 1 banana, peeled
- ¼ cup honey
- A pinch of salt
- 4 cups Greek yogurt

Directions:

1. Place all ingredients in a food processor. Pulse until smooth.
2. Turn on the Hamilton Beach and pour in the mixture.
3. Churn for 10 minutes.
4. Transfer in an airtight container and freeze overnight.

Nutrition Info: Calories per serving: 97; Protein: 3.2g; Carbs: 16.2g; Fat: 2.8g Sugar: 13.3g

Mango Texas Toast Ice Cream Sandwich

Servings: 2
Cooking Time: 15 Min
Ingredients:

- 1 loaf of Texas Toast bread (thick slices)
- organic honey to pour atop
- 1 mango (peeled & sliced)

Directions:
1. Toast your Texas Toast in a toaster. It should be nice and firm and golden brown.
2. Spread some of the mango slices on top of your Texas Toast.
3. Squeeze out and drizzle honey over both inside pieces of the Texas Toast.
4. Add a scoop of Ice Cream (that you made from this book) between the two pieces of Texas Toast and Enjoy!

Agave Lemon Chocolate Sorbet

Servings: 3
Cooking Time: 5 Hours
Ingredients:

- 2 cups water
- 1 cup unsweetened cocoa powder
- 3/4 cup agave
- 2 tablespoons lemon juice

Directions:
1. NOTE: Freeze your ice cream bowl for at least 24hrs prior to starting!
2. Mix together the water and agave in a medium saucepan on medium heat. Stir frequently until the agave dissolve. Mix in the cocoa powder and lemon juice and let the mixture come to a simmer. Let the

mixture cook for 3 minutes. Allow the mixture to cool completely. Then refrigerate covered for 2 hours.
3. Pour the ingredients into your ice cream maker, and let it churn for 25-30 minutes.
4. Place in an airtight container for up to 2 hours, until desired consistency is reached.

Summer Sorbet

Servings: 6
Cooking Time: 15 Minutes
Ingredients:

- 2 pounds fresh fruit of your choice
- 8 ounces sugar
- ¼ cup lemon juice
- ¼ cup vodka

Directions:
1. Place all ingredients in a blender. Pulse until smooth.
2. Place in the fridge and allow to chill for at least 3 hours.
3. Turn on the Hamilton Beach and pour in the mixture.
4. Churn for 10 minutes.
5. Transfer in an airtight container and freeze overnight.

Nutrition Info: Calories per serving: 268; Protein: 0.8g; Carbs: 67.4g; Fat: 0.8g Sugar: 54.6g

Feta Frozen Yogurt

Servings: 6
Cooking Time: 10 Minutes
Ingredients:

- 1 cup plain Greek yogurt
- ½ cup feta cheese
- 1 tablespoon honey

Directions:
1. Place all ingredients in a food processor. Pulse until smooth.
2. Turn on the Hamilton Beach and pour in the mixture.
3. Churn for 10 minutes.
4. Transfer in an airtight container and freeze overnight.

Nutrition Info: Calories per serving: 161; Protein:7 g; Carbs: 12g; Fat: 10g Sugar: 11g

Fun Fig Mint Milkshake

Servings: 6
Cooking Time: 25 Minutes
Ingredients:

- 2 cups heavy cream
- 1 cup milk
- 3/4 cup sugar
- 2 teaspoons vanilla extract
- 1/4 cup lemon juice
- 2 cups peeled, diced figs
- 2 teaspoons chopped fresh mint

Directions:

1. Refer to note at the beginning of the chapter about freezing bowl.
2. Place the milk and cream in a bowl, and mix them together until well combined. Use a whisk to mix in the sugar. Continue to whisk for about 4 minutes until the sugar dissolves. Then mix in the vanilla extract, lemon juice, and mint.
3. Pour the ingredients into your ice cream maker, and let it churn for 10-15 minutes, until desired consistency is reached. About 5 minutes before the ice cream is done churning add the figs to your ice cream maker.
4. Serve immediately.

Cinnamon Maple Bacon Milkshake

Servings: 6
Cooking Time: 25 Minutes
Ingredients:

- 2 cups heavy cream
- 1 cup milk
- 3/4 cup sugar
- 1 teaspoon cinnamon
- 1 teaspoons vanilla extract
- 6 slices finely chopped cooked thick cut bacon
- ½ cup maple syrup

Directions:

1. NOTE: Freeze your ice cream bowl for at least 24hrs prior to starting!
2. Place the milk and cream in a bowl, and mix them together until well combined. Use a whisk to mix in the sugar. Continue to whisk for about 4 minutes until the sugar dissolves. Then mix in the vanilla extract, cinnamon and maple syrup.
3. Pour the ingredients into your ice cream maker, and let it churn for 10-15 minutes, until desired consistency is reached. About 5 minutes before the ice cream is done churning add the bacon to your ice cream maker.
4. Serve immediately.

Black Raspberry Clementine Sorbet

Servings: Makes 1 Quart
Cooking Time: 4 Hours 35 Minutes
Ingredients:

- 20 chilled, peeled, and segmented clementine's
- ½ cup Black Raspberries
- 1 cup sugar
- ¼ teaspoon salt

Directions:

1. NOTE: Freeze your ice cream bowl for at least 24hrs prior to starting!
2. Use a food processor or blender to puree the Clementine's and black raspberries. Strain the puree until you have 4 ½ cups of juice. Place the juice and sugar back in the blender or food processor. Process until sugar dissolves. Then pulse in the salt until combined.
3. Pour the ingredients into your ice cream maker, and let it churn for 25-30 minutes.
4. Place in an airtight container for up to 2 hours, until desired consistency is reached.

Vegan Ridiculous Raspberry Coconut Frozen Yogurt

Servings: 1 Quart
Cooking Time: 2 Hours 35 Minutes
Ingredients:

- 2 cups coconut yogurt

- 1/4 cup sugar or maple syrup
- 1/2 teaspoon vanilla extract
- 1/4 cup shredded coconut
- ½ cup raspberries

Directions:

1. Refer to note at the beginning of the chapter about freezing bowl.
2. Puree the raspberries in a food processor or blender.
3. Place the yogurt in a bowl. Use a whisk to mix in the sugar. Continue to whisk for about 4 minutes until the sugar dissolves. Then mix in the vanilla extract, and raspberry puree.
4. Pour the ingredients into your ice cream maker, and let it churn for 25 minutes. About 5 minutes before the ice cream is done churning add the shredded coconut to your ice cream maker.
5. Put the frozen yogurt in an airtight container and place in the freezer for at least 2 hours, until desired consistency is reached.

Caramel & Pistachio Milkshake

Servings: 6
Cooking Time: 25 Minutes
Ingredients:

- 2 cups heavy cream
- 1 cup milk
- 1 cup brown sugar
- 1 teaspoon vanilla extract
- 2 ounces caramel
- 1/3 cup finely chopped pistachios
- 1 tablespoon butter

Directions:

1. NOTE: Freeze your ice cream bowl for at least 24hrs prior to starting!
2. Melt the butter in a small skillet on medium heat. Add the Pistachios, and cook for about 5 minutes, until they become lightly browned.
3. Place the milk and cream in a bowl, and mix them together until well combined. Use a whisk to mix in the sugar. Continue to whisk for about 4 minutes until the sugar dissolves. Then mix in the vanilla extract.

4. Pour the ingredients into your ice cream maker, and let it churn for 10-15 minutes, until desired consistency is reached. About 5 minutes before the ice cream is done churning add the caramel to your ice cream maker.

Tart Frozen Yogurt

Servings: 4
Cooking Time: 10 Minutes
Ingredients:

- 2 cups plain yogurt
- 2 cups plain Greek yogurt
- ¾ cup sugar
- 2 tablespoons honey
- Fruits for topping

Directions:

1. Place the yogurt, sugar, and honey in a bowl. Whisk to combine everything. Place in the fridge to chill.
2. Turn on the Hamilton Beach and pour in the mixture.
3. Churn for 10 minutes.
4. Transfer in an airtight container and freeze overnight.
5. Top with your favorite fruit before serving.

Nutrition Info: Calories per serving: 362; Protein: 21g; Carbs: 61g; Fat: 3g Sugar: 60g

Aromatic Earl Grey Tea Ice Cream

Servings: 6
Cooking Time: 2 Hours 50 Minutes
Ingredients:

- 2 cups heavy cream
- 1 cup milk
- 3/4 cup sugar
- 1 teaspoon vanilla extract
- 4 tablespoons earl grey tea

Directions:

1. Refer to note at the beginning of the chapter about freezing bowl.
2. Put the milk in a pan and bring it to a simmer. Add in the tea, take the pot off the heat, and allow to

seep for 5 minutes. Discard the tea, and allow milk to cool.

3. Place the milk and cream in a bowl, and mix them together until well combined. Use a whisk to mix in the sugar. Continue to whisk for about 4 minutes until the sugar dissolves. Then mix in the vanilla extract.

4. Pour the ingredients into your ice cream maker, and let it churn for 25 minutes.

5. Put the ice cream in an airtight container and place in the freezer for around 2 hours. Allow the ice cream to thaw for 15 minutes before serving.

Sweet Pumpkin Gingerbread Frozen Yogurt

Servings: 1 Quart
Cooking Time: 2 Hours 35 Minutes
Ingredients:
- 1 quart container full-fat plain yogurt
- ¼ teaspoon salt
- 1 cup sugar
- 1 teaspoon vanilla extract
- 1/2 cup pumpkin
- 2 tablespoons molasses
- 1 teaspoon cinnamon
- ¼ teaspoon ginger

Directions:
1. Refer to note at the beginning of the chapter about freezing bowl.

2. Place all the ingredients in a blender and blend on high until pureed and sugar dissolves.

3. Pour the ingredients into your ice cream maker, and let it churn for 25 minutes. About 5 minutes before the ice cream is done churning add the chocolate to your ice cream maker.

4. Put the frozen yogurt in an airtight container and place in the freezer for at least 2 hours, until desired consistency is reached.

Matcha Ice Cream

Servings: 6
Cooking Time: 2 Hours 50 Minutes

Ingredients:
- 2 cups heavy cream
- 1 cup milk
- 3/4 cup sugar
- 1 teaspoon vanilla extract
- 1 tablespoon matcha

Directions:
1. Refer to note at the beginning of the chapter about freezing bowl.

2. Place the milk and cream in a bowl, and mix them together until well combined. Use a whisk to mix in the sugar. Continue to whisk for about 4 minutes until the sugar dissolves. Then mix in the vanilla extract. Finally whisk in the matcha until well mixed.

3. Pour the ingredients into your ice cream maker, and let it churn for 25 minutes.

4. Put the ice cream in an airtight container and place in the freezer for around 2 hours. Allow the ice cream to thaw for 15 minutes before serving.

Pumpkin Frozen Yogurt

Servings: 4
Cooking Time: 10 Minutes
Ingredients:
- 2 cups plain Greek yogurt
- 4 ounces low-fat cream cheese, softened
- ½ cup canned pumpkin, mashed
- ¼ cup brown sugar
- 1 tablespoon pumpkin pie spice
- 1 teaspoon vanilla extract

Directions:
1. Place all ingredients in a food processor. Pulse until smooth.

2. Turn on the Hamilton Beach and pour in the mixture.

3. Churn for 10 minutes.

4. Transfer in an airtight container and freeze overnight.

Nutrition Info: Calories per serving: 198; Protein:12 g; Carbs: 24g; Fat: 7g Sugar:20 g

Strawberry English Muffin With Honey Ice Cream Sandwich

Servings: 2
Cooking Time: 15 Min
Ingredients:

- 1 pack of English muffins
- organic honey to pour atop
- small pack of strawberries

Directions:
1. Toast your English muffins in a toaster just like you would for breakfast.
2. Spread about 4-5 strawberries on top of your warm muffin.
3. Squeeze out and drizzle honey over both inside pieces of the English muffin.
4. Add a scoop of Ice Cream (that you made from this book) between the two pieces of English muffins. Enjoy!

Vegan Chocolate Soft Serve Ice Cream

Servings: 9
Cooking Time: 50 Minutes
Ingredients:

- 3/4 cup water
- 1 1/4 cups full fat coconut milk or coconut cream (as thick as possible)
- 2/3 cup organic cane sugar
- 2/3 cup unsweetened cocoa powder
- 1/4 tsp sea salt
- 6 ounces vegan dark chocolate, finely chopped
- 1/2 tsp pure vanilla extract

Directions:
1. Refer to note at the beginning of the chapter about freezing bowl.
2. Put the first 5 ingredients in a large saucepan, and heat it on medium-high heat. Mix the ingredients together using a whisk. Allow the mixture to come to a low boil. Continue to whisk often, and remain cooking on a low boil for 1 minute.
3. Take the pan off the heat, and mix in the chocolate and vanilla extract using the whisk. Continue to mix until the chocolate is melted.

4. Place the mixture in a blender, and blend on high speed for about 30 seconds.
5. Allow the mixture to cool
6. Pour the ingredients into your ice cream maker, and let it churn for 25 minutes.
7. Serve immediately.

Lemon Mint Melon Sorbet

Servings: 4
Cooking Time: 3 Hours 10 Minutes
Ingredients:

- ½ cup lemon juice
- 1 cup boiling water
- 1 cup chopped mint
- ½ cup melon
- Zest of 1 lemon
- 1 cup sugar

Directions:
1. NOTE: Freeze your ice cream bowl for at least 24hrs prior to starting!
2. Mix together the sugar, lemon zest, mint and melon in a heat safe bowl. Then pour in the water, and stir frequently until sugar dissolves. Let the mixture sit for 20 minutes. Then strain it into another bowl. Mix in the lemon juice and let the mixture cool totally.
3. Pour the ingredients into your ice cream maker, and let it churn for 25-30 minutes.
4. Place in an airtight container for up to 2 hours, until desired consistency is reached.

Lemon Lime Soda Milkshake

Servings: 6
Cooking Time: 25 Minutes
Ingredients:

- 2 cups heavy cream
- 1 cup milk
- 3/4 cup sugar
- 1 teaspoon vanilla extract
- ¼ cup lime juice
- ¼ cup lemon juice
- ¼ cup 7up or Sprite

- Zest of one lemon
- Zest of one lime

Directions:

1. NOTE: Freeze your ice cream bowl for at least 24hrs prior to starting!
2. Place the milk and cream in a bowl, and mix them together until well combined. Use a whisk to mix in the sugar. Continue to whisk for about 4 minutes until the sugar dissolves. Then mix in the vanilla extract, juice, Sprite/7-Up and zest.
3. Pour the ingredients into your ice cream maker, and let it churn for 10-15 minutes, until desired consistency is reached.
4. Serve immediately.

Directions:

1. First, make sure you preheat oven to 345 degrees F. Take the sugar cookie dough and make them into 1 tablespoon balls and place them on the parchment baking sheet paper. Put them in the oven and bake till lightly golden brown
2. Approximately 10 minutes.
3. Let the cookies cool for about 5 minutes on baking sheets
4. You can then move them to wire rack to cool.
5. Once cool, place giant scoop of ice cream onto one cookie and sandwich with another cookie on top. Roll in lightly crushed candy canes and freeze for about 30min.

Peach Frozen Yogurt

Servings: 5
Cooking Time: 10 Minutes

Ingredients:

- 4 cups fresh peaches
- 3 tablespoons honey
- ½ cup plain Greek yogurt
- 1 teaspoon vanilla extract

Directions:

1. Place all ingredients in a food processor and pulse until smooth.
2. Turn on the Hamilton Beach and pour in the mixture.
3. Churn for 10 minutes.
4. Transfer in an airtight container and freeze overnight.

Nutrition Info: Calories per serving: 109; Protein: 3g; Carbs: 24g; Fat: 3g Sugar: 23g

Candy Cane Ice Cream Sandwiches

Servings: 6
Cooking Time: 35 Minutes

Ingredients:

- 1 lb. Sugar cookie dough
- vanilla ice cream
- Crushed candy canes
- Sprinkle of cinnamon

Lime-mango Sorbet

Servings: 8
Cooking Time: 15 Minutes

Ingredients:

- ½ cup water
- ¼ cup sugar
- 5 cups ripe mango cubes
- 1 teaspoon lime zest
- ¼ lime juice

Directions:

1. Place sugar and water in a saucepan. Bring to a boil until the sugar dissolves.
2. Remove from the heat and place in the fridge to chill for at least 3 hours.
3. Place all ingredients in a blender and add the chilled sugar mixture. Pulse until smooth. Allow to chill for another two hours.
4. Turn on the Hamilton Beach and pour in the mixture.
5. Churn for 10 minutes.
6. Transfer in an airtight container and freeze overnight.

Nutrition Info: Calories per serving: 88; Protein: 1g; Carbs: 22g; Fat: 1g Sugar: 19g

Aromatic Rose Gelato

Servings: 4-6

Cooking Time: 2 Hours 35 Minutes

Ingredients:

- 1/2 cup heavy cream
- 2 cups milk
- 3/4 cup sugar
- 1 teaspoon rose extract

Directions:

1. Refer to note at the beginning of the chapter about freezing bowl.
2. Place the milk and cream in a bowl, and mix them together until well combined. Use a whisk to mix in the sugar. Continue to whisk for about 4 minutes until the sugar dissolves. Then mix in the rose extract.
3. Pour the ingredients into your ice cream maker, and let it churn for 25 minutes.
4. Put the gelato in an airtight container and place in the freezer for up to 2 hours, until desired consistency is reached.

Lime Sorbet

Servings: 7

Cooking Time: 15 Minutes

Ingredients:

- 2 cups water
- 1 cup sugar
- 4 limes, zest
- Juice from 8 limes

Directions:

1. Place the water and sugar in a saucepan. Bring to a boil until the sugar dissolves.
2. Remove from the heat and place in the fridge to chill for at least 3 hours.
3. Turn on the Hamilton Beach and pour in the water-sugar mixture, lime zest, and lime juice.
4. Churn for 10 minutes.
5. Transfer in an airtight container and freeze overnight.

Nutrition Info: Calories per serving:74 ; Protein: 0.3g; Carbs: 20.6g; Fat: 0.1g Sugar: 13 g

Orange Sorbet

Servings: 7

Cooking Time: 15 Minutes

Ingredients:

- 1 orange, zest, and juice
- 2 cups water
- 1 1/3 cups sugar
- 3 cups fresh orange juice
- 4 tablespoons lemon juice

Directions:

1. Place all ingredients in a saucepan. Turn on the heat and allow to simmer for 5 minutes or until the sugar dissolves.
2. Remove from the heat and place in the fridge to cool for 2 hours.
3. Turn on the Hamilton Beach and pour in the mixture.
4. Churn for 10 minutes.
5. Transfer in an airtight container and freeze overnight.

Nutrition Info: Calories per serving: 146; Protein: 1g; Carbs: 35.9g; Fat: 0.2g Sugar: 30.6g

Caribbean Pineapple Mint Sorbet

Servings: 9

Cooking Time: 2 Hours 40 Minutes

Ingredients:

- 1 diced, peeled, and cored small pineapple
- 2 tablespoons lemon juice
- ½ cup mint
- 1 cup plus 2 tablespoons sugar

Directions:

1. NOTE: Freeze your ice cream bowl for at least 24hrs prior to starting!
2. Puree the pineapple, mint and lemon juice in a food processor or blender. Then add in the sugar and puree until the sugar dissolves.
3. Pour the ingredients into your ice cream maker, and let it churn for 25-30 minutes.
4. Place in an airtight container for up to 2 hours, until desired consistency is reached.

Mango Pineapple Sorbet

Servings: 6
Cooking Time: 10 Minutes
Ingredients:
- 1 cup fresh ripe mango, peeled and cubed (seed removed)
- 1 cup pineapple tidbits
- ¼ cup water
- 1 teaspoon lemon juice
- ½ cup sugar
- ½ teaspoon salt

Directions:
1. Place all ingredients in a blender. Pulse until smooth.
2. Place in the fridge to chill for 2 hours.
3. Turn on the Hamilton Beach and pour in the mixture.
4. Churn for 10 minutes.
5. Transfer in an airtight container and freeze overnight

Nutrition Info: Calories per serving:74 ; Protein: 0.4g; Carbs: 19g; Fat: 0.1g Sugar: 10g

Chocolate Matcha Gelato

Servings: 4-6
Cooking Time: 2 Hours 35 Minutes
Ingredients:
- 1/2 cup heavy cream
- 2 cups milk
- 3/4 cup sugar
- 1 teaspoon vanilla extract
- 1 tablespoon matcha
- 2 ounces chopped dark chocolate

Directions:
1. Refer to note at the beginning of the chapter about freezing bowl.
2. Place the milk and cream in a bowl, and mix them together until well combined. Use a whisk to mix in the sugar. Continue to whisk for about 4 minutes until the sugar dissolves. Then mix in the vanilla extract. Finally whisk in the matcha until well mixed.

3. Pour the ingredients into your ice cream maker, and let it churn for 25 minutes. About 5 minutes before the ice cream is done churning add the chocolate to your ice cream maker.
4. Put the gelato in an airtight container and place in the freezer for up to 2 hours, until desired consistency is reached.

Blueberry Frozen Yogurt

Servings: 6
Cooking Time: 10 Minutes
Ingredients:
- 2 ½ cups blueberries, fresh or frozen
- 2/3 cup honey
- 1 small lemon, zested and juiced
- ¼ teaspoon salt
- 2 cups full fat yogurt, chilled

Directions:
1. Place all ingredients in a food processor. Pulse until smooth.
2. Turn on the Hamilton Beach and pour in the mixture.
3. Churn for 10 minutes.
4. Transfer in an airtight container and freeze overnight.

Nutrition Info: Calories per serving: 262; Protein:5.12 g; Carbs: 61g; Fat: 1.6g Sugar: 58.9g

Ice Cream Pizza

Servings: 8
Cooking Time: 30 Minutes
Ingredients:
- 1 cup cold whole milk
- ¾ cup granulated sugar
- 2 cups cold heavy cream
- 1 teaspoon vanilla extract
- 1 commercial pizza dough, cooked according to package instructions
- 5 pieces Oreo cookies, crushed
- ½ cups M&Ms, chopped
- ½ cup hot fudge sauce

Directions:

1. Put ice water in a large mixing bowl. Place a small bowl on top of the large bowl with ice. Pour cold milk and sugar into the small bowl and whisk until the sugar is dissolved. Stir in the cream and vanilla. Stir to combine.

2. Place the cold freezer bowl in the Hamilton Beach Ice Cream Maker. Turn on the machine and pour in the mixture. Add one package of crushed Oreos five minutes before the time ends.

3. Stop in 25 minutes until the mixture becomes soft and creamy.

4. Transfer into an air-tight container and freeze overnight.

5. Spread ice cream in a dough and top with Oreo cookies and M&Ms. Drizzle with hot fudge sauce.

6. Slice and serve.

Nutrition Info: Calories per serving:387 ; Protein: 11g; Carbs: 35.9g; Fat: 22.7g Sugar: 19.8g

Luscious Lavender Sour Cherry Sorbet

Servings: 6
Cooking Time: 5 Hours 35 Minutes
Ingredients:
- 3 cups pitted, sliced sour cherries
- ½ teaspoon lavender
- 3/4 cup sugar
- 1/2 teaspoon salt
- 2 tablespoons vanilla extract
- 2 ½ teaspoons lime juice

Directions:
1. Refer to note at the beginning of the chapter about freezing bowl.

2. Use a food processor or blender to puree the lavender, sugar, cherries, and vanilla extract. Then blend in the salt and lime juice. Strain the mixture into a bowl, and refrigerate covered for 2-3 hours.

3. Pour the ingredients into your ice cream maker, and let it churn for 25-30 minutes.

4. Place in an airtight container for up to 2 hours, until desired consistency is reached.

Passion Fruit Sorbet

Servings: 8
Cooking Time: 15 Minutes
Ingredients:
- 1 cup boiling water
- ¾ cup sugar
- 8 passion fruit, flesh scooped
- Juice from 1 lemon

Directions:
1. Place water and sugar in a saucepan. Bring to a boil until sugar dissolves. Remove from heat and allow to chill in the fridge for at least 2 hours.

2. While the sugar syrup is chilling, place the passion fruit in a blender and pulse until smooth. Pass the mixture into a sieve to remove the seeds. Discard the seeds and save the juice.

3. Mix the passion fruit juice with the sugar syrup and add the lemon juice.

4. Turn on the Hamilton Beach and pour in the mixture.

5. Churn for 10 minutes.

6. Transfer in an airtight container and freeze overnight.

Nutrition Info: Calories per serving:55 ; Protein: 0.4g; Carbs: 13.9g; Fat: 0.2g Sugar: 6g

Rhubarb Ice Cream Cake

Servings: 16
Cooking Time: 35 Minutes
Ingredients:
- 4 stalks fresh rhubarb, chopped
- 1 medium gala apple, chopped
- ½ cup water
- 1 cup raspberries
- ½ cup white sugar
- 1 cup cold whole milk
- ¾ cup granulated sugar
- 2 cups cold heavy cream
- 1 teaspoon vanilla extract

Directions:
1. Place in a bowl the rhubarb, apple, water, raspberries, and sugar. Boil over medium flame and

simmer for 10 minutes. Drain and set aside in the fridge. Reserve the juices.

2.   In a bowl, mix together the graham crackers and butter to form a dough. Press dough in spring form pan and place in the fridge to chill.

3.   Put ice water in a large mixing bowl. Place a small bowl on top of the large bowl with ice. Pour cold milk and sugar into the small bowl and whisk until the sugar is dissolved. Stir in the cream and vanilla. Stir to combine.

4.   Place the cold freezer bowl in the Hamilton Beach Ice Cream Maker. Turn on the machine and pour in the mixture. Add one package of crushed Oreos five minutes before the time ends.

5.   Stop in 25 minutes until the mixture becomes soft and creamy.

6.   Place in a spring form pan and top with the chilled fruit sauce.

Nutrition Info: Calories per serving: 121; Protein:1.22 g; Carbs: 13.8g; Fat: 7.3g Sugar: 12.2g

Cherry Mango Sorbet

Servings: 2
Cooking Time: 15 Minutes
Ingredients:

- 1 cup frozen mango chunks
- ½ cup frozen pineapple chunks
- 1 cup preserved cherries
- 1 tablespoon water

Directions:

1.   Place all ingredients in a blender. Pulse until smooth.

2.   Turn on the Hamilton Beach and pour in the mixture.

3.   Churn for 15 minutes.

4.   Transfer in an airtight container and freeze overnight.

Nutrition Info: Calories per serving:202 ; Protein: 1.7g; Carbs: 51.7g; Fat: 0.3g Sugar: 32g

Apple Chocolate Gelato

Servings: 4-6

Cooking Time: 2 Hours 35 Minutes
Ingredients:

- 1/2 cup heavy cream
- 2 cups milk
- 3/4 cup sugar
- 1 teaspoon vanilla extract
- 1 cup apples
- ½ cup finely chopped semi-sweet chocolate

Directions:

1.   NOTE: Freeze your ice cream bowl for at least 24hrs prior to starting!

2.   Puree the apples in a food processor or blender.

3.   Place the milk and cream in a bowl, and mix them together until well combined. Use a whisk to mix in the sugar. Continue to whisk for about 4 minutes until the sugar dissolves. Then mix in the vanilla extract and apple puree.

4.   Pour the ingredients into your ice cream maker, and let it churn for 25 minutes. About 5 minutes before the ice cream is done churning add the chocolate to your ice cream maker.

5.   Put the gelato in an airtight container and place in the freezer for up to 2 hours, until desired consistency is reached.

Vegan Radical Raspberry Chocolate Soft Serve Ice Cream

Servings: 9
Cooking Time: 50 Minutes
Ingredients:

- 3/4 cup water
- 1 1/4 cups full fat coconut milk or coconut cream (as thick as possible)
- 2/3 cup organic cane sugar
- 2/3 cup unsweetened cocoa powder
- 1/4 tsp sea salt
- 6 ounces vegan dark chocolate, finely chopped
- 1/2 tsp pure vanilla extract
- 1/2 cup raspberries

Directions:

1.   Refer to note at the beginning of the chapter about freezing bowl.

2. Put the first 5 ingredients in a large saucepan, and heat it on medium-high heat. Mix the ingredients together using a whisk. Allow the mixture to come to a low boil. Continue to whisk often, and remain cooking on a low boil for 1 minute.

3. Take the pan off the heat, and mix in the chocolate and vanilla extract using the whisk. Continue to mix until the chocolate is melted.

4. Place the mixture in a blender with the raspberries, and blend on high speed for about 30 seconds or until the raspberries are pureed.

5. Allow the mixture to cool

6. Pour the ingredients into your ice cream maker, and let it churn for 25 minutes.

7. Serve immediately.

Chili Lime Mango Sorbet

Servings: 6-8
Cooking Time: 2 Hours 40 Minutes
Ingredients:
- 3 peeled, pitted, and diced large mangos
- 2 cups simple syrup
- 1/4 cup fresh lime juice
- 1 tablespoon chili powder
- Pinch of salt

Directions:
1. NOTE: Freeze your ice cream bowl for at least 24hrs prior to starting!

2. Puree the mangos in a food processor or blender. Then add in the remaining ingredients and blend on low until combined.

3. Pour the ingredients into your ice cream maker, and let it churn for 25-30 minutes.

4. Place in an airtight container for up to 2 hours, until desired consistency is reached.

Walnut Mint Pomegranate Frozen Yogurt

Servings: 1 Quart
Cooking Time: 2 Hours 35 Minutes
Ingredients:
- 1 quart container full-fat plain yogurt
- ¼ teaspoon salt
- 1 cup sugar
- 1 tablespoon mint extract
- 1 cup 100% pomegranate juice
- 1/2 cup walnuts

Directions:
1. NOTE: Freeze your ice cream bowl for at least 24hrs prior to starting!

2. Place the yogurt in a bowl. Use a whisk to mix in the sugar and salt. Continue to whisk for about 4 minutes until the sugar dissolves. Then mix in the mint extract, and pomegranate juice.

3. Pour the ingredients into your ice cream maker, and let it churn for 25 minutes. About 5 minutes before the ice cream is done churning add the chocolate chips to your ice cream maker.

4. Put the frozen yogurt in an airtight container and place in the freezer for at least 2 hours, until desired consistency is reached.

Mint Greek Frozen Yogurt

Servings: 10
Cooking Time: 10 Minutes
Ingredients:
- 3 cups plain Greek yogurt
- 1 cup sugar
- ¼ cup lemon juice
- 2 teaspoons vanilla
- 1/8 teaspoon salt
- 2 tablespoons mint, chopped finely

Directions:
1. Place the yogurt, sugar, lemon juice, vanilla, and salt in a cold bowl. Whisk until smooth. Add the chopped mint.

2. Turn on the Hamilton Beach and pour in the mixture.

3. Churn for 10 minutes.

4. Transfer in an airtight container and freeze overnight.

Nutrition Info: Calories per serving: 84; Protein: 2g; Carbs: 15g; Fat: 1g Sugar: 5g

Peach Mango Frozen Yogurt

Servings: 5
Cooking Time: 4 Minutes
Ingredients:
- 1 ½ cups Greek yogurt
- 1 cup sliced peaches
- 1 cup diced mango
- ½ cup sugar
- 1 teaspoon vanilla extract

Directions:
1. Place all ingredients in a food processor. Pulse until smooth.
2. Turn on the Hamilton Beach and pour in the mixture.
3. Churn for 10 minutes.
4. Transfer in an airtight container and freeze overnight.

Nutrition Info: Calories per serving: 182; Protein: 14.8g; Carbs: 31g; Fat: 1g Sugar:29 g

Honey Cinnamon Blackberry English Muffin Ice Cream Sandwich

Servings: 2
Cooking Time: 15 Min
Ingredients:
- 1 pack of English muffins
- organic honey to pour atop
- small pack of blackberries
- 1 tsp. cinnamon

Directions:
1. Toast your English muffins in a toaster just like you would for breakfast.
2. Spread about 4-5 blackberries on top of your warm muffin.
3. Squeeze out and drizzle honey over both inside pieces of the English muffin.
4. Sprinkle a little cinnamon on top
5. Add a scoop of Ice Cream (that you made from this book) between the two pieces of English muffins. Enjoy!

APPENDIX : RECIPES INDEX

CPSIA information can be obtained
at www.ICGtesting.com
Printed in the USA
LVHW061520300721
693916LV00006B/549

9 781801 662239